THE HEALTH ODYSSEY

From Myths to Mindsets

BELLA VERD

THE HEALTH ODESSEY
Copyright © 2024 by neurodivergent

Contents

CHAPTER
1

Part 1

Beyond the Plate:
The Importance of Holistic
Health for a Vibrant Life

"People killin', people dyin'
Children hurtin', I hear them cryin'
Can you practice what you preach?
And would you turn the other cheek?
Father, father, father help us
Send some guidance from above
'Cause people got me, got me questionin'
Where is the love?"
–*"Where Is The Love?" by Black Eyed Peas.*

think this pretty grim song is best suited for what I am about to tell you.

Sarah had been struggling with health issues, particularly weight gain, for many years. To lose some of her weight she had tried every kind of diet; from a low-fat diet to a low-carb diet. She also had spent so many hours at the gym every week, but nothing seemed to be working for her. Sarah felt like giving up as she was utterly frustrated and exhausted.

One day, on her way home from work, she craved a quick snack, so she popped into a coffee shop and opted for a granola bar thinking that it was much better and "healthier" than those cupcakes and pastries on display. As she chewed away the granola bar, she noticed that it had a surprisingly sweet taste,

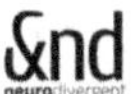

even though she clearly remembered reading the label which stated that it contained only natural sugars. She immediately flipped the package over and read the ingredients of the snack. Immediately her heart sank when she discovered that this "healthy" snack was loaded with preservatives, artificial flavors, and even processed sugars.

Sarah sat down on the chair by the window, staring at the granola bar in her hand. This was a wake-up call for her as she realized that even when she thought she was making healthy life choices, she was being tricked by the food industry which made her consume junk food. And as a result of being led astray by the misleading labels, not only her physical but her mental health suffered a lot as well.

She looked at the counter and noticed a guy in his stationary jog, wearing his running gear, with his smartphone on his arm using an armband, and wiping the sweat off of his upper lip. He took one of his air pods out and asked the person behind the counter for the same granola bar that Sarah had just gotten. It made Sarah feel worse and better at the same time.

Worse because it was really alarming how common this trickery in the food industry was. She realized that the food is often engineered for maximum profit rather than maximum health. This is why we are bombarded with messages that tell us what to eat, but these messages rarely have any science or common sense behind them. This is exactly the reason people have conflicting points of view regarding what healthy diets should and should not contain, and also a cause of many chronic diseases due to the number of processed foods consumed.

Better because there was hope for Sarah. All the struggle that she had gone through, the mental breakdowns, and the hopelessness that she could never get healthy was not her fault at all. She realized that she needed to be the one in control of

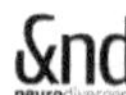

her health now and it would start with questioning the labels, learning to cook from scratch, and seeking out natural foods. This would help her body and mind to heal and achieve the health goal and vitality that she deserves. With this thought, Sarah got up and went out of the coffee shop with a huge smile on her face and handed out the granola bar to the homeless person sitting just outside the coffee shop.

"I'm putting my foot down!"

Something somewhat similar to what happened with Sarah happened to me too. You see, I had always been skeptical of what I consume daily. So one casual day I was in a grocery store, going through only those aisles that had fresh produce, lean proteins, and whole grains, and avoiding the aisles holding processed foods and packaged snacks. I was feeling pretty good about my diet choices, and I couldn't wait to go home and prepare a nice healthy home-cooked meal from scratch – I even had the perfect recipe that I was excited to try.

I picked up a box of wholegrain cereal for my breakfast on working days when I am usually in a rush. It was by chance that I turned the box over and read the ingredients. Noticing how the "whole grain" cereal was loaded with processed sugars. I looked around a bit and discovered that the "all-natural" snacks were packed with preservatives and artificial sugars. And worst of all, the "green juices" lacked actual vegetables and were all sugars.

Boy was I frustrated and defeated! A healthy diet was a lot more complicated than I had expected. But I wasn't going to give up easily. I went home and did some research on how I could make actually healthy choices in a world that seemed determined to promote unhealthy ones. During my research, I did figure out one thing, the challenges of diet in the modern world are real – no doubt, but so are their solutions. One of

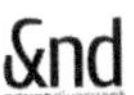

the solutions is to start taking responsibility for your own well-being and demand a food system that prioritizes health over profit.

Let's get real here for a minute. The food we put into our bodies matters. A lot. It's not just about satisfying our cravings or filling our stomachs. It has a direct relation to our health and our well-being. And if we are not making healthy and wise choices, we are in trouble. If you still didn't understand the mechanism behind it, let me dumb it down for you: our bodies are just like machines. When we put fuel in a machine, it starts to work, and the fuel is what keeps them running. If you are constantly filling up your body with processed foods, snacks, and sugary drinks, and all that junk, you're not really giving the nutrients that your body actually needs.

I can't emphasize it enough; by eating processed foods and these unhealthy snacks, you are depriving your body of the building blocks that are needed to make healthy cells, energy, and power for your muscles and brain. In fact, you're loading up on calories which will only contribute to your weight gain and in some cases, chronic diseases.

When you provide your body with the whole, natural foods that it needs, you're getting access to vitamins, minerals, healthy fats, and clean sources of proteins. These are the tools your body requires to thrive. These foods give you energy that lasts long, as compared to the quick bursts of energy you would get from sugars that leave you crashing and burning. Moreover, your immune system, your gut health, and your mental clarity, all of it is supported and augmented in ways that can significantly improve your quality of life.

It's not just about what you eat. It's also about your habits, your lifestyle, and how you eat. In one scenario if you are constantly snacking, or eating while sitting – or worse, lying – in front of

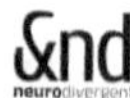

the TV, or munching while mindlessly scrolling through social media on your phone, you are going to be overweight due to all the overeating you're doing subconsciously. Because of your laziness, you are not giving yourself the chance to your body to fully and properly digest the food and on top of it you are not being aware of the fullness cues and hunger.

On the other hand, if you make your mealtime kind of like a sacred ritual, taking time to set the plates, paying attention to how your body feels before, during, and after the meal, and actually savoring the food, then you – my friend – have created a positive relationship with food. This is going to lead you to make more informed decisions and choices and because of this, you will know what your body truly needs and how different foods make you feel.

Now, I know what you're thinking, "But Muneeba, I am too busy! I don't have time to make informed food choices!" Hey, trust me I get it. The world we live in is a hectic, demanding, and fast-paced one. But the fact of the matter is that making informed food decisions doesn't have to be complicated or time-consuming. In fact, it is actually quite simple. You just have to understand the basics of nutrition and then use that understanding to make the choices for you. Now, this doesn't mean that you become experts in the field of nutrition, it just means that you need to apply that learned knowledge willingly, bit by bit to your daily life.

For instance, you don't have to make elaborate meals, consuming hours in the kitchen. You can make simple dishes with just a few ingredients. You also don't have to give up your favorite treats entirely. Instead, indulge in moderation. If you are adding your treat onto your plate then make sure that the plate isn't completely full of that treat, and also make sure that that the plate is balanced out with plenty of whole foods and healthy, nutrient-rich products.

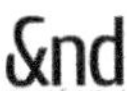

Let me make it relatable for you. Earlier, when I was in the grocery store, feeling frustrated about the cereal box and the misleading information, I came up with strategies during my research that would help me make better food choices without consuming much of my time. First and foremost, I started reading the labels very carefully. I looked for ingredients that I recognize and want in my diet, and I avoid the products containing ingredients that I don't want like added sugars, artificial flavors, and preservatives. Secondly, I started focusing on whole foods and unprocessed foods, and believe me this was one of the best ways to keep my body healthy when I have to prepare meals from scratch, it keeps my mind fresh as the whole process of cooking is really therapeutic. And lastly – this one is for people like me who have weak moments every now and then – I completely avoid the aisles that have junk foods and unhealthy snacks and processed foods.

It is as simple as that.

As soon as I started practicing these strategies, I realized that making healthy choices was so easy and manageable. Now, I feel more confident and can enjoy a good, tasty meal without worrying about what it's going to do to my health. I mean, sure it is not going to be easy at the start. Heck, I even remember one of my colleagues bringing a box of donuts. I never craved a donut as much as I did that day. But I had to be strong and steadfast and was not going to let Karen and her donuts sabotage my efforts.

All right, now let's talk about the elephant in the room: the misinformation and various food myths. It feels like wherever we look, we have a magical superfood or a new fad diet that is going to solve all our health issues in a miraculously short period of time. Let me tell you right now that this is all BS.

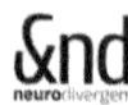

To be honest, fad diets lack scientific justifications and evidence, and this is why my book is going to cut through the noise and nonsense and provide you with research-based information that you can trust to be accurate and safe. You know, there are some pretty pervasive food myths out there like the importance and the humane need to detox your body using juice cleanses, and that all kinds of carbs are bad. Let's not forget the infamous diet trends that take you to the extreme, like keto and paleo. These are some of the myths that you need to debunk in order to have an actual healthy dietary regimen.

The bottom line is: making informed food decisions is one of the most impactful and powerful actions you could take for your health and well-being. This awareness should never be about short-term feelings, it's about setting yourself up for a long, healthy, and vibrant life.

Take time to educate yourself, and experiment with different foods and habits. And the most important thing is to be kind to your body. Your health will thank you.

So, are you ready to take control of your health and start living a more vibrant life? Let's do this.

Part 2

Dieting Dangers: The Truth About Fad Diets

Fad diets. *Ugh*. I don't even like the sound of it. What kind of a word is 'fad'? If you come across something called a 'fad' diet and *still* decide to follow it, well there is no hope for you then, my friend. These are the diets that promise you quick and easy weight loss, improved health, boosted immune system, and a myriad of other health benefits. You've probably heard of them all: keto, paleo, juice cleanses, and whatnot. But allow me to tell you that the reality of fad diets is far from the hype.

Simply put, fad diets are trending extreme diet plans that promise dramatic results. These are also known (and better termed) as restrictive diets because these require the elimination or restriction of an entire food group. They do provide rapid weight loss in a short period of time, but they fail to provide the necessary nutrients that are vital for long-term health.

I get it. It seems like a dream to have a quick fix, but at what cost? Having conversations about fad diets with someone who believes in them has made me realize the misconceptions they have. Allow me to shatter those misconceptions so that you may have a clearer perspective.

First of all, the fact that these diets are an easier and quicker fix is totally false. They not only drop your weight all of a sudden but also deprive you of the essential nutrients and minerals

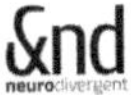

that your body requires. How is this a fix? If at first, all you had to deal with was your weight issues, then now you're going to have to deal with weight issues *and* dehydration, malnutrition, heart problems, etc.

Second of all, these diets are far from sustainable. You can't keep these up for your whole life. Whenever there are ups and downs in your health, you have to change your diet according to your needs. If you are sticking to one diet, you are increasing the risks of falling ill, and when you slip off of the diet plan, you not only regain the weight you lost but also some more. And the health issues still remain there. Do you honestly think that if you stick to these kinds of diets, you will magically get into perfect health and physique? Come on!

Third of all (yes there is a third of all), one of the most dangerous false claims of these fad diets is that people really believe them to be harmless Just because these diets are famous and popular all over social media, doesn't mean that they are totally safe for you. Many of the fad diets lead to severe nutrient deficiencies, malnutrition, dehydration, organ damage, and even death. And I'm not being dramatic.

Oh, and one more misconception that people have about the fad diets is that these are "natural" and "cleaner" diets. Wrong. These fad diets make you think you are having a "cleaner" meal by removing the "harmful" food group. This is where the problem lies. There are no "bad" or "harmful" food groups! Everything – even fats – can play a healthy role as a component in your diet if added in moderation.

Food is not the enemy!

I am sick of hearing the statement that carbs are the enemies. Carbohydrates are one of the most essential sources of energy in our bodies and cutting this food group out is definitely going

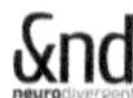

to invite a whole bunch of health problems. Add complex carbs to your diet like the ones in fruits and vegetables and whole grains and stay energized throughout the day. Moreover, people have been talking trash about fats since forever. I mean, the idea that fat is bad for you is completely outdated. I know you have been hearing this a lot that low-fat diets are the key to a healthy and long life, but this is not true at all. In fact, many authentic studies have shown that the healthy fats in nuts, olive oil, avocados, etc., are so beneficial for you that these fats actually lower the risks of heart diseases and improve brain activity and functioning.

And because I am beyond annoyed with the constant stream of misinformation and dangerous advice that is being peddled in the name of "health" and "wellness" I want to take a moment and explain what these diets are.

Keto – The Diet That Puts the 'Die' in 'Diet'

One of the most popular fad diets is the ketogenic, or simply keto diet. The restrictive eating pattern revolves around low-carb and high-fat design. This is supposed to put your body in a state of ketosis, which is when the body burns the fat for fuel, instead of carbohydrates (which we are depriving the body of). Another similar fad diet is the Atkins diet. It basically follows the same low-carb and high-fat approach, but it differs from the keto diet in a way that the carbohydrate intake in the Atkins diet is gradually increased.

Okay, sure, both of these diets might lead to some weight loss in the short term, but at what cost? The high amounts of fat in this diet can be responsible for some serious health problems like heart disease, and on top of it, the lack of carbohydrates can result in nutrient deficiencies. Oh and don't even get me started on how difficult it is to stick to it in the long term. Can you imagine not having carbs for the rest of your life? If

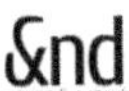

you slipped up and gave in to your cravings you may actually end up regaining the weight you lost and more, how about that? People who have sworn by this diet never tell you what happens in the long run.

Paleo – Embrace the Nutrient Deficiencies of Our Ancestors!

The Paleo diet is another one of these restrictive diets. When I heard about this diet, I could actually understand how it could make sense for some of you. But then I went ahead and did some research of my own, instead of believing what was written in the article. This Paleo diet gets its name due to the Paleolithic era. People believe that if we eat like our ancestors from the said era, we will be happier and healthier. First off, this notion alone, that our ancestors were healthier and happier than us, is ridiculous. I mean people in that era were hunter-gatherers. Which means that they had to hunt for food. The harsh environment, the extreme weather, the dangerous predators, the limited food sources, long periods of famine, and food scarcity, which of these features makes you think that our ancestors were healthy and happy? Secondly, we have access to modern medicine and nutrition sciences now. We don't need to survive on just selective food groups. The Paleo diet restricts grains, dairy, and processed foods and promotes the consumption of only meats, vegetables, and fruits. Again, sure, it sounds like a good idea to avoid processed foods, but restricting dairy and whole grains is taking it too far. Don't even get me started on the nutritional deficiencies this can cause. I don't need to tell you that calcium and vitamin D are really vital for your health. Are you really willing to sacrifice your overall health and well-being just to follow some fad diet that's based on a romanticized view of the past?

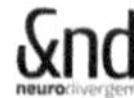

Juice cleanse – Drink Your Way to Malnutrition

Another popular fad diet is the juice cleanse. Even the name implies how extreme this diet is. This diet promises quick weight loss but delivers nothing but harm. You have to drink fruit and vegetable juices for several days, typically ten, or even weeks, and nothing else. This might seem like a healthy way to 'cleanse' your body, but it's just another one of the ways to deprive your body of essential nutrients all the while messing up your digestive system. The irony is that this particular restrictive diet is aimed at giving your digestive system a break.

Trust me when I say this: there is no evidence that states that juice cleanses are effective for anything, well, except for depriving your body of the essentials. Juice cleanses, no doubt, will give you the rapid weight loss it promised but have some common sense and think: you would be starving yourself (hence the weight loss). And don't even get me started on the lack of protein, fiber, and healthy fats in these juices which can lead to muscle loss, digestive tract issues, and other health problems. And let's not forget about the blood sugar spikes from all that fruit juice.

HCG Diet – Because Your Body Needs More Hormones, Obviously

Next up on our list is the HCG diet. HCG is the human chronic gonadotropin hormone that is produced during pregnancy I swear, how do people even come up with these? This fad diet is one of the most controversial ones and involves injecting HCG following a very low-caloric diet. You may know by now that a very low-calorie diet leads to muscle loss and nutrient deficiencies, and the injection of hormones can have serious health risks.

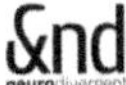

Why do people keep falling for these, is the million-dollar question. Are people so desperate for a quick fix that they are willing to risk their health for a shortcut?

Diets that help you "Drop a Dress Size" – More like "Drop Unconscious During the Day"

The paleo, the keto,
The trendy diets of the day,
They promised her beauty,
But led her to decay.

A girl tried keto, she thought it was right,
But soon her health took a terrible plight.
Ketosis took hold, her body in shock,
Till death overtook, a tragic block.

So let this be a warning,
To those who would be swayed,
By the false promises of fad diets,
And the prices they've already paid.

–Me

I might not be a member of the Black Eyed peas but maybe I should be. Anyway, do you remember Sarah? Well, After her incident with the coffee shop granola bar, she was still optimistic and determined to maintain her health and physique despite her busy schedule. She decided to investigate various exercise routines and fad diets. She even considered hiring a personal trainer to help her achieve her goal.

One day, during her research, she stumbled upon an article that was about this magical new diet plan. The article's headline was something like this: "Drop a Dress Size in a Week with This

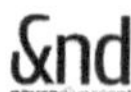

Simple Diet". Because Sarah had a job that demanded long hours and she had a really hectic routine, she was immediately intrigued by the bold claims and decided to give it a try. The diet required Sarah to cut out entire food groups and severely restrict her calorie intake. It basically consisted of eating only protein and vegetables and eliminating all carbohydrates and fats from her diet.

At first, she felt amazing. She was feeling good, her weight was rapidly decreasing, and she felt a huge sense of accomplishment. However, after some time, she started having a different kind of experience. She felt lethargic, severely fatigued, experienced horrible headaches and even fainting spells. Her mind was so convinced that this diet is good for her, that she blamed all these new feelings and conditions on her stress from work. She started to feel like her work is taking a toll on her health.

Things took a turn for the worse when one day Sarah was out for a jog, and suddenly she collapsed. Her body was rushed to the hospital where, after tests and diagnosis, it was concluded that Sarah was severely dehydrated and malnourished. Unfortunately, her body was in a state of shock due to the extreme dieting and her health was in serious jeopardy. As she lay in the hospital bed, she realized what she had done to her body. She realized that she had been chasing an unrealistic ideal and that the restrictive diets she had tried had only caused harm to her body and mind.

Searching answers on the internet about what went wrong with her health and diet, she came across a statement by Dr. Jane Smith, a registered dietician and nutrition consultant stating, *"Fad diets may provide a quick fix, but they often lack the essential nutrients our bodies need to thrive. It's important to focus on a balanced, sustainable approach to nutrition that includes a variety of foods and doesn't involve extreme deprivation."*

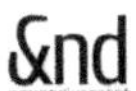

Sarah realized that she had been so obsessed with achieving her body goals that she completely compromised her health and well-being. She knew that these fad diets are neither sustainable nor healthy. Lucky for her, she still had some hope and willpower. She did not accept that she would be weak and wanted to find the best way to regain her health and also maintain her weight. The money she had spent on a personal trainer, was now being spent on a nutritionist who took responsibility to plan out her diet and exercise routine. She learned the importance of listening to her body and nourishing it with whole, nutrient-dense foods.

The case of Oprah Winfrey helped motivate her further. Oprah Winfrey was also struggling with fad diets. Over the years, she has tried various diets, including the liquid diet, where she consumed only liquids for several weeks. This led to a rapid weight loss of 67 pounds, but also caused her health issues like dizziness and weakness. Oprah later admitted that the diet was not sustainable and that she regained the weight as soon as she returned to regular eating habits. She now advocates for a balanced approach to nutrition and has publicly discussed her journey toward finding a healthier relationship with food.

Slowly but surely, Sarah began to feel like a new person. She had more energy, felt more confident in her body, and was able to enjoy the simple pleasures of life, like going out to eat with friends and family. She no longer felt like she had to deprive herself in order to be healthy.

There are so many women and girls who unfortunately get caught and stuck in this whirlpool of fad diets. Let me share a real-world example with you which took the media by a storm.

This is the story of a 21-year-old girl named Eloise Aimee Parry. In 2017, Eloise came upon an online supplier in the UK who sold these magical pills that would help her lose weight in an

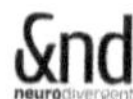

unbelievably short amount of time. It is totally understandable how tempting these pills were for young girls struggling with weight loss can be. Moreover, these pills were described as "fat-burning" chemicals. Parry ingested 8 of these pills and within hours she experienced severe side effects like rapid heartbeat, difficulty breathing, high fever, and vomiting.

These pills, which were illegally marketed as a weight loss product, actually contained an industrial chemical called 2,4-dinitrophenol, or DNP for short. This highly toxic chemical is used for the manufacturing of explosives. Despite the fact that she was immediately rushed to the hospital, she couldn't survive, and she died several hours later.

Look, I get it. We all want to find that one magical diet that will solve all of our problems and make us feel amazing. But here's the truth: there is no such thing. These cases are cautionary tales for those who believe that there is a quick fix to achieve health and happiness. The truth is that the path to a healthy life is a lifelong journey that requires patience, perseverance, and a commitment to self-care. The idea that there is some "perfect" diet out there that will work for everyone is complete nonsense.

And yet, I have seen so many people falling for these myths. It especially makes me so aggravated when they jump from one fad diet to another, and then onto the next, hoping that *this* time the diet will work. One time, it'll be them going vegan, the other time it'll be them drinking nothing but juices for a whole week, and the next time it'll be them cutting out carbs when they should actually stop and think about their decisions and its effects on their health.

What's worse is that these kinds of fad diets wrap you in a cycle of deprivation and bingeing. You might be able to stick to your diet for a while but sooner or later your body will start to rebel. You will crave the very foods that your body has been deprived

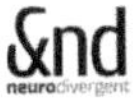

of. Eventually, you will give in to your cravings. And when you do, you might go for overeating. This will lead to guilt and shame, and you will fall back to the restrictive diet plan. These fad diets will spin you back and forth between deprivation and bingeing just like a yo-yo.

It is so important to understand that food is not the enemy here. Our bodies demand a varied and balanced diet that is not falling into the one-size-fits-all genre. Different people might have different needs. Karen from HR might need to stop eating all those donuts, but pale, thin, and quiet Kyle from IT can eat one or two. It's all about incorporating all food groups in moderation and finding what works best for you. The concept is all about moderation.

Listen! Balance, not Deprivation.

I can't emphasis enough on this. Let me simplify it for you. When you cut out entire food groups from your diet, you basically deprive your body of the nutrients that it needs in order to function properly. This lack of nutrients can lead to deficiencies, weakened immune systems, and many other health problems.

The one simple solution for all this is creating a balance, not deprivation. Opting for a balanced approach to nutrition means that you're eating a whole variety of foods from all the food groups but in moderation. And – before you ask – yes it does include carbs, fats and even sugars. Mostly these include plenty of fruits, vegetables, lean proteins, and whole grains.

You can't have a balanced approach for two weeks and then go back to your old ways. This is a lifestyle change that required dedication and commitment. So to sum it up I have written a step-by-step guide as to what you need to do:

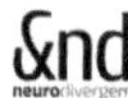

1. Let go of the idea that there is a 'perfect' diet out there.
2. Make sure you add moderate amounts of foods to your diet from each and every food group.
3. Listen to your body and figure out what's best for you. It could mean that you need a more plant-based meal. Or it could also mean that you need a little bit more fat in your diet. Keep in mind that there is no one-size-fits-all approach here.
4. Make this your lifestyle.

At the end of the day, what's best for your body is what matters the most. So the next time you stumble upon a fad diet promising some miracle, as yourself if this quick, risky, and suspicious fix is what your body actually needs instead of a moderate and balanced approach to nutrition. I'll answer this one for you: no, your body certainly does not need this quick fix. It's time to prioritize our health over a temporary fix. It's time to break free from the dictated diet culture and start focusing on your body's needs by embracing a balanced approach. Trust me, your body will thank you for it.

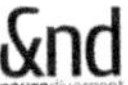

CHAPTER
2

Part 1

Cracking the Culinary Code: Separating Fact from Fiction

I can understand if you are feeling a bit confused now. I can feel what's probably going on in your mind. Heck, I can practically hear the question, "But Muneeba, where to start for achieving this 'balanced approach' you talk about?"

You sound just as muddled as Sarah.

After her recovery from the fad diet consequence, she couldn't help but feel accountable for every little inconvenience regarding her health. If she didn't have a good sleep, she would wonder if she had consumed any sugars. If she had a stomachache, she would unintendedly make it worse by stressing about what she had eaten wrong. This was a never-ending cycle of skeptical thoughts, and once Sarah went down the rabbit hole, coming back took longer than it should.

Getting fed up, she decided to do some research again, but this time it was more like a 'truth-finding' mission, rather than research. She looked for all those myths that the internet and even the big companies have us believing. And boy, was she baffled. What she found out was truly as if she had been deceived her whole life.

Sometimes it's essential to approach with a healthy dose of skepticism.

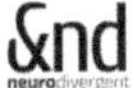

In a world of food fables, where myths are spun,
I rise up to expose them, one by one.

That's exactly what we are going to do right now because it is time that I put an end to these misguided beliefs, so take mental notes as we separate fact from fiction.

Carbophobia Exposed

Myth # 1: *"Carbohydrates make you fat"*

If I had a penny for every time I heard a "diet enthusiast" talk about this, I'd be chillin' in my mansion right now. The tale of carbohydrates and their supposed role in weight gain has been going on for far too long. The truth is that weight gain is not exclusive to carbs only. Weight gain sneaks in when we gain an excess amount of calories, no matter the food group they are obtained from. Now before you get all *factual* on me, allow me to give you some scientific justification. This will probably make you understand carbs better and I hope your relationship with them is mended.

So, there are two basic kinds of carbohydrates in foods, okay? One of them are known as simple carbs, or 'refined carbs'. And the other group is known as complex carbs. The terms simple and complex are appointed on the basis of the structure of the carbohydrate. I have even added a structure comparison for you so you may visualize what I'm talking about. You can clearly tell which of these are the refined carbs and which ones are the complex carbs. Obviously, the one on the right is a complex carb that, I don't even think it has a name. Whereas the one on the left is sweet little glucose.

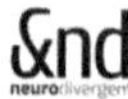

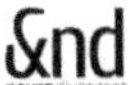

Simple carbohydrates are present in white bread, white rice, pastries, pasta, white flour – you get the idea, whereas the complex carbs are found in fruits, beans, oatmeal, barley, whole grain bread, whole grain cereals - basically whole plant foods. Now - stay with me - simple carbohydrates make you gain weight. These have a simple structure, and they digest rapidly, which is why one feels like they can have another serving. And this leads to overeating, and eventually weight gain.

However, complex carbs do not cause weight gain at such a pace. This class of carbohydrates are not calorie dense – usually. I mean, yes there are always some exceptions but the categories and examples I've mentioned are not involved in weight gain. Just be mindful of your serving size.

Fat Liberation

Myth # 2: *"Fats are always bad for you"*

Oh, this one is followed and believed *so* blindly that I can't even begin to express how much it bothers me. The way carbs are of two types, good and bad, similarly, fats also have good and bad categories. We have saturated fats, and then we have unsaturated fats. Our friend is the unsaturated fat. Let me break this one down for you as well, scientifically.

Saturated fats - are also known as trans fats, or trans fatty acids - are "saturated" with hydrogen atoms, no double bonds in their chemical structure. This means that they can easily change their state of matter and hence, are able to solidify at room temperature.

Keeping this in mind, if you consume such fats that are going to solidify later on, imagine how clogged your arteries would be. But if you consume the right kind of fat from the right source in the right amount, you have nothing to worry about.

You need to set the record straight now. You have the necessary knowledge of the chemistry of these saturated and unsaturated fats. Consume the good kind of fat in moderation and you will not gain pounds. With that in mind, let's address another common confusion.

Fat or cholesterol; which one to blame?

Whenever I come across this particular myth, I feel obligated to educate and inform about the difference between fats and cholesterol. Cholesterol is a much more complex version of fat (or fatty acid). Have a visual below and you'll see how complex cholesterol molecule (on the right) is as compared to a simple fatty acid (glycerol, on the left).

Cholesterol also has two categories: High density lipoprotein (HDL) and Low density lipoprotein (LDL). Answer me this, if the LDL tends to remain in the arteries, and HDL tends to go into the liver for further metabolism, which one is the bad cholesterol? Yep, you guessed it right; the one that stays in

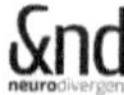

your arteries. This might lead to clogged arteries and vessels, and eventually heart problems.

For the purpose of avoiding consumption of bad cholesterol and saturated fatty acids, work on finding the foods that are a source of HDL and / or unsaturated fatty acids. For your lazy self, I have mentioned a few examples:

A list of the foods containing saturated fats:

- Beef, pork, poultry, any animal meat basically.
- Certain plant oils like coconut oil (you must have seen how coconut *oil* is solid at room temperature)
- Some dairy products like cheese, butter etc.
- Processed meats like sausages and bacon
- Pre-packed snacks like pastries, cookies, chips etc.

And here is a list of the foods containing unsaturated fats:

- Nuts
- Plant oils
- Certain fish meat that contains omega-3 unsaturated fatty acids like salmon, tuna.
- Olives
- Avocados

Just remember, your body needs the good cholesterol for the protection of nerves and the production of various necessary structures like hormones.

Protein for All!

Myth # 3: *"Protein is only for body builders"*

If you are someone who avoids consumption of proteins, thinking that you don't need them in your diet as you are

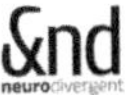

not a bodybuilder, well, not much can be done about you, except that I try my best. I'm going to take more of a biological approach to this, rather than a chemical one.

Listen, your whole body's muscles are made up of proteins. The skeletal muscles attached to your skeleton, responsible for movement: protein. The cardiac muscles, like the ones in your heart, which are responsible for pumping blood nonstop since before you were even born: protein. The smooth muscles that make up the actual structure and internal linings of organs (like the gut): protein!

How is it possible to think that you don't need them, until you want to gain muscle mass? This nutrient is NOT just for the gym enthusiasts. We need the protein as our muscles get tiny tears and repairs quite often.

Yes I understand the point of view of the fitness freaks. They exercise to build muscle mass and because the proteins are building blocks of muscles, they consume diets and foods loaded with proteins. I'm sure you must have heard of someone who swallowed raw eggs for the sake of protein. Ew.

Incorporating lean sources of proteins like fish, poultry, legumes, tofu, lentils in your meals is crucial for muscle support, growth and overall wellbeing. Remember that!

Milk Monopoly

Myth # 4: *"Dairy is essential for strong bones"*

This one is not as extreme as the others, but I needed to address this for you too. First of all, keep this piece of information forever in your mind: vitamin D, physical activities and a balanced nutritional diet are equally important for bone

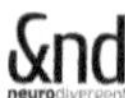

health. That being said, let's talk about milk. We have all heard the saying *'milk does the body good'*. True: milk is definitely one of the excellent natural sources of vitamins, and minerals, particularly calcium. However, milk (or particularly cow milk) isn't the only option for getting these nutrients. We have fortified plant-based milk (like almond milk) available in the market – if you're vegan. Other than that leafy green vegetables like broccoli and kale are also great sources of calcium. There is never just one kind of option, you have just got to explore a bit.

A 'Berry' Sweet Misconception

Myth # 5: *"All fruits are equal"*

You have no idea how common this misconception is among people, that they can eat just about any fruit and get the same nutritional value, because -according to them - all fruits have the same variety of essential vitamins and minerals in them?!

Generally, fruits are considered as a rich source of vitamins, minerals and fibers. But some fruits stand out for a particular benefit, or nutrient group. Take berries for example: they are loaded with antioxidants that will fight inflammation in the body, boosting the immune system and also improve brain health by protecting the neural network, and eventually prevent age-related memory loss. Citrus fruits are another great example of fruits known for their vitamin C immunity booster. You get the gist, each fruit brings its own set of unique roles, so it is essential to consume a diverse food platter, of course in moderation. I am eating some berries right now actually.

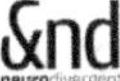

Night Owl Nourishment

Myth # 6: *"Eating late at night causes weight gain"*

Ah, this brings me to my childhood, when my grandmother would poke my belly and scare me that all those meals after 8 pm would give me a muffin top. Good ol' days. The infamous "no eating after 8" is such a hype, so let's set the record straight for once and for all. Starting from the basics: weight gain occurs when you consume more calories than you require. This fact is regardless of the food group, and regardless of the time of the day. Problem occurs with the mindless snacking and the tasty yet unhealthy munching. Most people would never consume fruits or vegetables when they're watching a late night movie. They would always go for snacks, and it's always the unhealthy ones. Your digestive system is bound to cry and be upset when you stuff your gut with cheeseburgers and pizzas at night. You, however, can now enjoy a healthy meal any time hunger strikes.

Organic Obsession

Myth # 7: *"Organic food is always healthier"*

I might get some disagreement, but this needed to be said. Someone *had* to say it. It seems like everywhere I turn; I am bombarded with messages and advertisements about the superiority of organic foods, and how they are far better and healthier than the normal food grown conventionally.

I understand the fame, I get the hype. But the way a product is grown, or the environment that a product has been provided for growth doesn't make up the nutritional content and the health benefit of that product.

Just to be clear, I am not saying that organic foods are worse, or that they should not be used. And I do know that organic

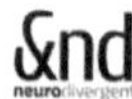

farming has its benefits, I simply mean that the myth that organic food is *healthier* than the produce's conventionally grown counterparts is nothing but a myth.

The Hunger Myth

Myth # 8: *"Skipping meals is a surefire way to lose weight"*

The allure of skipping meals in order to shed a few pounds has always been the strongest force and most commonly opted way. But let me open your eyes to the bitter truth; this omission of meals can actually work against you. Depriving your body pf the natural nourishment and the required nutrients will lead to you having an increased hunger, developing a habit of overeating and will result in a slowed-down metabolism.

If you do manage to lose some pounds after skipping meals, then you have lost anything but fat because fats actually take more energy to break and hence they are the last ones be utilized by the body, body's proteins (muscle mass) being the first – as carbs are not provided due to the skipped meal.

Imagine the dangers you may put your body through: weakened immune system, unhealthy digestive system, fatigue and light headedness, etc. Just do me a favor and listen to your body. Focus on portion control, balanced meals, and your body's hunger and fullness cues.

Fat and Fabulous

Myth # 9: *"'Low fat' or 'fat-free' is always a healthier choice"*

I know we just debunked the myths and misconceptions regarding the fat group, but I felt like this 'fat-free' label needed its own attention. The label 'low fat' has led us to

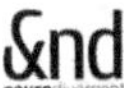

believe that this is a healthier option. Let me enlighten you: when manufacturers remove fat from food products, they most often compensate for it with artificial ingredients, added sugars and various other unhealthy additives that make up for the lost flavor.

Fats are vital for the normal metabolism of the body, but if you still want to avoid fat, do me a favor and start to avoid the 'fat-free' or 'low-fat' labelled products as well. You do know that you can always opt for a healthier option when it comes to fats, right?

The Great Detox Deception

Myth # 10: *"Detox diets flush out the toxins"*

These detox trends: they promise to cleanse our bodies of all the alleged toxins that are lurking within. Listen to mee carefully; our bodies are equipped with a natural, highly efficient detoxification system – the liver and the kidneys. These restrictive diets, the juice cleanses, are nothing but a marketing tact for the benefit of the industry, not the consumer.

I feel the need to deliver another biology lesson here. It is always important to understand the scientific evidence and justification before hopping on the bandwagon. Have a look at the filtration system of kidneys. The body's fluid goes through 3 filtration units in the kidney: through the glomerulus – which is the basic filtration apparatus, through the tubules – passively diffusing the easy-to-remove toxins, and through the tubules again – but actively this time, to forcefully get rid of the not-so-easy-to-remove toxins. Liver has a whole other mechanism. It consists of a massive army of phagocytic immune cells who are ready to eat the toxins quite literally. You need to just focus on nourishing the bodies, let our bodies decide how, when and what to naturally get rid of.

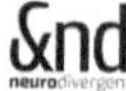

The stream of food myths is never-ending, and it is time to bid farewell to these misconceptions. These myths are enough to make your blood boil! It's just simply frustrating to see these baseless myths persist and continue to mislead naïve people like you. My only intention was to shed light on what truly constitutes a healthy and balanced approach to nutrition, as you had asked me at the start of this chapter, remember? So take a moment to pause and reflect. Keep in mind that you are always supposed to question these myths because in this battle against these food misconceptions, knowledge is our only weapon. Leave no stone unturned.

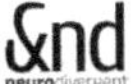

Part 2

The Poster Child
of Modern Food Culture:
Processed Food

Doesn't it feel liberating to finally feel relieved of the burden of confusion and oblivion regarding the food misconceptions? Don't get too comfortable because I want to talk about another culinary villain: processed food.

Ah, they're everywhere, aren't they? From the colorful aisles in the supermarket to the carefully organized and stacked shelves in the convenience stores, these processed foods have managed to infiltrate every nook and cranny of our lives. The come with this false promise of instant gratification and they fool people like you with their cunning tactics. But let me tell you the dark truth behind the bright flashy packaging: processed foods are the embodiment of all that is wrong with our food choices.

If you do not know what processed foods are, well let me dumb it down for you. Anything that has chemicals, or is canned, or dehydrated, is a processed food. More or less. Not only do these processed foods contain artificial flavors, but they also contain a number of mysterious chemicals that wreak havoc on our health and lead to chronic diseases and obesity. Their most common trick: convenience. They make us believe that we are saving time and effort.

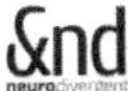

How unfortunate that we have become so accustomed to these processed products, that er have forgotten what real food tastes like. It's like they've cast a spell over our senses, making it impossible to appreciate the subtle joys of fresh produce and whole grains. I mean, who needs the vibrant colors and flavors of nature when you can have artificially enhanced mediocrity? Our bodies cry for nourishment because we have settles for these empty calories and artificial substitutes. Let's just call it what it is; processed foods are imposters of the culinary world, lacking any real nutritional value and being the root cause of our dietary downfall, all the while masquerading as a convenient solution.

Now, in today's fast-paced world, I get how convenience can take precedence over health. I mean, it sounds so easy and effortless when we realize that processed foods offer a quick fix for our hunger, and our taste buds can be satisfied with amazing flavors. However, once you realize the consequences, you will lose your appetite.

Allow me to break it down for you. You see, one of the most concerning aspects of these processed foods are the presence of a high level of unhealthy fats, sugar, and sodium. These three ingredients, or as I like to call them – appropriately so – as *the Deadly Trio*, are notorious for the detrimental effects on our health. You are not unperceptive of the unhealthy fats that I have mentioned here. These are present in abundance, and these have always been the leading cause of obesity, heart diseases and various other chronic disorders. The high sodium intake leads to high blood pressure, fluid retention and heart problems, and the sugar consumption increases the risk of diabetes, and dental problems.

Heart disease, diabetes, cancer, mental health disorders – you name it, these types of foods are just waiting to serve it up on a greasy platter.

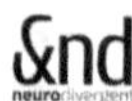

The Unholy Trinity: Sugar, Fat and Salt

Processed foods are the epitome of nutritional disappointment. Not only do these products deceive us and lack essential nutrients, but they also actually have the audacity to leave us undernourished in spite of the calorie bursts that they provide. It's like they're playing a cruel game of hide-and-seek with our bodies, withholding the very things we need to thrive.

I'm just going to give it to you straight; the main culprits are these food companies. They have always exploited our weakness for their own profit. These food companies are aware of the fact that if they load their food products with salt, sugar or fat, our taste buds will have the time of their life and crave more. And this eventually leads us down a path of never ending cycle of cravings and overconsumption that fill their pockets. This unholy trinity are, as Michael Moss in "Salt, Sugar and Fat" would call them, the company jewels. And let's not forget about the marketing shenanigans that these companies pull off. The way these products seem to have a "scientific justification" behind them, makes us get manipulated and sucked into their devious tactics. They know exactly what they are doing, and they do not care about the consequences.

Master the Art of Label Reading – A Guide to Navigating the Aisles

That is where I come in. I am about to share what knowledge and information I have gathered regarding the deadly trio and many other processed food ingredients, and when you will realize how bad these processed foods are for your health, you'll get infuriated and will question the moral compass of these companies.

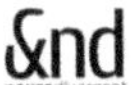

I am talking about the complicated ingredient list including various substances like high fructose corn syrup, refined grains, trans fats and many others that you can't even pronounce. Prepare yourself for an unsettling journey into the dark heart of processed foods where every bite is addictive and seasoned with betrayal. For visuals, how about you imagine you and I are walking through the aisles of a grocery store, picking up food products and reading the labels.

1. Palm oil

"Break free from its greasy grasp"

Trans fats are produced when regular fats like corn, palm oil etc., are bombarded with hydrogen and made into a solid state. The purpose of making fats into trans fats is only for the sake of preservation. Which basically means that the packaged food will stay 'fresh' for a longer period of time, and it can stay on the shelves of the store or supermarket for many years without spoiling or going bad. These trans fats can increase the bad cholesterol in your blood and meanwhile lower the good cholesterol as well. Avoid these trans fats like palm oil and also bid farewell to fried food too because these items are fried using the trans fatty oils.

2. Shortening

"The Unhealthy Shortcut to Flavor and Texture"

If you read the ingredients list and you see shortening, or partially hydrogenated oil as one of the ingredients, ditch that product immediately. Shortening is also one of the types of trans fats and they offer the same health risks as the unhealthy fats. You know, I have always wondered why it is known as shortening and I am sure you must be wondering that too. Turns out, it is called that because of its property to shorten the gluten fibers in the dough. If gluten fibers are not shortened, it will produce a dough that

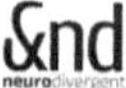

stretches, like the one we prefer for pizza. But when we add shortening, it makes the overall product appear 'crumbly'. Butter is a good example of a shortening. It is always better to consume healthier fats like olive oil, canola oil etc.

3. White flour, white rice and white bread

"Out with the white, in with the right"

Whole grains have always been refined for the purpose of increasing and extending their shelf life but in the process of refining the product, the nutrients get sucked out and therefore there are no fibers, minerals and vitamins left for us. Moreover, these wholegrains, stripped out of their nutrients are a bit too easy to digest for the human gut, and hence we gain a lot less, even after eating a lot more. Not to mention the blood sugar level skyrocketing. Whenever you go grocery shopping, always prefer the whole grains instead of refined ones lie brown rice, oatmeal, whole wheat breads etc. These are the ones you need to consume. Just avoid the pale parade altogether, understand?

4. High fructose corn syrup

"The sticky sweet trap"

I cannot emphasize this enough that the mother of all refined sugars is high fructose corn syrup. In many processed food packaging, it is also abbreviated as HFCS. With the awareness of the harms of refined sugars, people have lowered their consumption. But the amount of high fructose corn syrup is now 20 times more abundant in our diet than the refined sugars. As per research, people consume more calories from high fructose corn syrup than any other food group or source. You should have a strict 'no tolerance' policy for this one because it is going to damage your health by boosting up fat storing hormones,

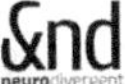

increasing cravings and overeating which eventually leads to weight gain.

5. Artificial sweeteners

"A bittersweet betrayal"

You should always scan the ingredient list of any product for artificial sweeteners and if it contains these substances then you immediately put that product back in the aisle. These artificial sweeteners may sound like aspartame, saccharin, sucralose etc. Now I have mentioned it numerous times that artificial sweeteners can cause weight gain through cravings, but I guess I have to explain it to you in order for you to fully understand the science behind it. You see, we have a mechanism in our brains that is known as *the food reward pathway*. In literally very simple words, when we taste these artificial sweeteners, our neurons release the pleasure hormone, dopamine. Because if this, the brain starts to connect that particular food with pleasure, hence developing a food reward pathway. This pathway ensures that the behavior will be repeated. In short, artificial sweeteners trick your brain into wanting to consume more of these processed foods and making you overeat and gain weight. Moreover, these artificial sweeteners lack calories (because they are not actually sugars)which means that due to these, our brain never really completes the activation of the food reward pathway, and we end up with unsatisfied cravings even if we have had a good amount of such snacks. It is definitely a bittersweet betrayal, isn't it?

6. Artificial colors

"Shades of Deception"

The word 'artificial' should be enough on its own to make you avoid consuming the product you're examining. Turn that brightly colored package around and look for names

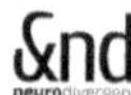

like Yellow #5 or Blue #1. These artificial colors, derived from petroleum and coal tar, are employed to make the food appear more appealing. But they've been linked to numerous health issues, including allergies, hyperactivity, and even cancer. The same goes for preservatives like BHA and BHT. These chemicals extend the shelf life of products but are suspected carcinogens and endocrine disruptors. Always remember, it's not just about how the food looks or lasts; it's about what it does to your body. If the ingredient list of processed foods contain artificial colors, then put the product back in the aisle and search for something more natural and color-free. Especially look out for these in products intended for consumption by children. They are responsible for a number of cancers like adrenal, bladder, brain, thyroid, kidney etc. You need to be serious about eliminating processed foods from your life because the consequences are too grim.

7. MSG

"Sweet, salty and sinister"

MSG, or Monosodium glutamate is a flavor enhancer that affects brain chemistry. It has been reported that MSG causes lesions in the brain that lead to many abnormalities of the cognitive, emotional or endocrinological systems. Now you might have heard that glutamates are present in natural foods as well, like cheese or meat, but let me clarify that the substances used by the food industry manufacturing these processed items use the technique hydrolysis to obtain free glutamates that are separated from their host proteins. You should definitely play it safe and always go for naturally flavored foods. You can even add natural flavors to spice your meal up like the good old-fashioned seasoning using various herbs and condiments, but I beg you to keep yourself and your loved ones away from these taste manipulators.

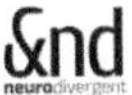

8. Preservatives

"From Shelf Life to Health Strife"

Sodium and potassium benzoates are added to processed foods for the purpose of preservation. The preservatives have the sole task of making sure that the product remains free of contamination, and it remains 'fresh' and stable for a longer period of time. This is what they call enhancing the shelf life. But little did you know that benzene is a known carcinogenic and is connected with some serious thyroid problems. Normally you would find such preservatives in soda bottles to make them safe from mold growth. The situation gets worse when these preservatives are combined with vitamin C or ascorbic acid, and when these plastic bottles are exposed to high temperature, benzene can accumulate in a dangerous amount, unsafe for use. Do not take such a risk and avoid these preservatives.

I can practically *hear* your confusion, "But Muneeba, if these preservatives are so harmful, how are they allowed? Isn't there anyone to keep a check on this?" The FDA is responsible for approving chemicals like preservatives. You'll be surprised to know that the FDA has some preservatives deemed safe, for instance BHA or Butylated Hydroxyanisole. It's a mouthful, I know. This particular preservative has the tendency to mess up your endocrine system, meaning that it causes imbalance of hormones when consumed. What's worse is that BHA is in hundreds of processed foods, and it comes with many aliases. You can either go on the internet and search the various disguises and names of BHA or you can simply avoid the hassle and ditch these processed foods altogether.

The preservatives normally found in processed meat like hot dogs and bacon, are sodium nitrates and sodium nitrites. No, this is not a typo. These are some of the worst ones. Thy cause metabolic disturbances on a level that

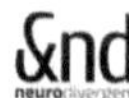

leads to chronic conditions like diabetes. They also have been known to cause colon cancer. Just do me a favor and protect your health from such chemicals.

9. Gluten

"Biological Rust to our Bodies"

Gluten is one of those ingredients that have been notorious for causing inflammatory responses in the body. And a lot of people are seen taking care of it if gluten causes them allergies or mild inflammatory responses. When I talk about inflammation, I am talking about the typical responses of the body's immune system *"whether it's the redness that quickly appears after an insect bite or the chronic soreness of an arthritic joint,"* as David Perlmutter states in Grain Brain. *"This typical body reaction creates swelling and pain as responses to stress, both of which are indicators of the inflammatory process."* Problems arise when inflammation gets out of control.

When inflammation spirals out of control, it leads to the production of chemicals that are directly harmful to our cells. This then causes a reduction in cellular function followed by cellular destruction. In Western societies, uncontrolled inflammation is prevalent, with research showing it to be a fundamental cause of diseases such as coronary artery disease, cancer, diabetes, Alzheimer's, and virtually every other chronic disease one can imagine.

Inflammation doesn't merely cause physical discomfort; it's closely linked to brain degeneration processes. In the heart of chronic inflammation lies oxidative stress - a form of biological rusting that happens to all tissues. Oxidative stress is essentially a by-product of our body's process of turning food and oxygen into energy. This natural process can become harmful if it goes rampant or if the body can't maintain it under control.

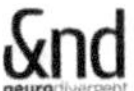

One particular player in oxidative stress is gluten, a protein that has a major role in causing brain inflammation. Gluten, which means glue in Latin, is a protein composite that binds flour together to make various bread products. However, gluten or its subcomponents could initiate an immune re-action, leading to inflammation, which is the cornerstone of many brain disorders. It's also worth noting that fat, specifically good fats like Omega-3s and monounsaturated fats, reduce inflammation, whereas modified hydrogenated fats commonly found in commercially prepared foods dramatically increase inflammation. I think I've convinced you enough for you to take care about the presence of gluten in your product's ingredient list.

Time to break free

It is essential to recognize what impact these processed foods have on your health and that the damage these would cause is an irreparable one. Don't worry, you can still navigate your way through the aisles and heal your body with healthy options. You just have to embrace a balanced and varied diet consisting of fresh, whole, unprocessed food items. Here's a tip, choose anti-inflammatory ingredients, like turmeric – which contains the active curcumin – and incorporate anti-inflammatory products in your life, like probiotics. It is time to break free from the clutches of these processed foods and we need to reclaim our tastes. We need to explore the vibrant world of the nutrients and flavors which are natural and authentic.

Consider this as a wakeup call.

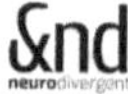

CHAPTER
3

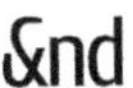

Part 1

Food Navigation 101: How to Win at Picking the Best Foods

Discovering the hidden dangers of processed foods was a wakeup call for Sarah as well. She made a habit of digging up the truth whenever she would come across anything remotely confusing or suspicious. The mental torture she went through in her life regarding food and diet had been traumatizing for Sarah and she always felt like she had to walk on eggshells when it comes to grocery shopping.

Initially she kept getting disappointed. Whenever she would step into her kitchen to unload the groceries, she would turn over the bottle or the package and read what was in it. Sarah felt like the grocery store was not the most practical place to take out her phone and go on the internet to discover what each ingredient is, hence, her habit of reading the labels once she got home. But the moment she would realize what she had actually bought, it would always leave her disappointed and frustrated.

All of this was too overwhelming for Sarah. She neither wanted a hovering, bright red question mark over her head while shopping, nor was she a fan of the distress her mind would go into when she found out what the ingredients actually are. And let's not discuss how guilty she felt when she would knowingly pick up a processed food item just for the sake of convenience

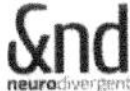

and time saving. But this was not as overwhelming as her state of health a few years back when she did not care what she was consuming, and all she could think about is where did all these extra pounds come from. But it was only a matter of time and determination that Sarah had discovered a way to win at this.

She cracked the code!

Sarah figured out a few strategies and tactics to overcome the challenge that she would face in the labyrinth of the grocery store where there was temptation to be found at every turn. With an overwhelming wave of exhilaration, she sat down at her desk and started to go through her previous notes. Yes, she kept notes - that's how dedicated she was to change her unhealthy habits. Anyway, she identified what were the critical control points of her shopping routine that needed to have a control preventative measure which would help her avoid the hazard of getting tempted and – regretfully so – buying processed and unhealthy food items.

Going through her notes, she felt the adrenaline rush as realization dawned upon her on every page she turned. In a fear of forgetting her newfound salvation, she jotted down the necessary key points that she most definitely needed to adapt while shopping for food. When she was done reviewing every page and had recalled all her purchasing habits, Sarah held in her hand the key to all her problems. A list of tactics and strategies to help her achieve healthy shopping and eventually healthy eating. She called it as *'Sarah's Smart Eating Strategies'* and it looked something like this:

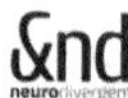

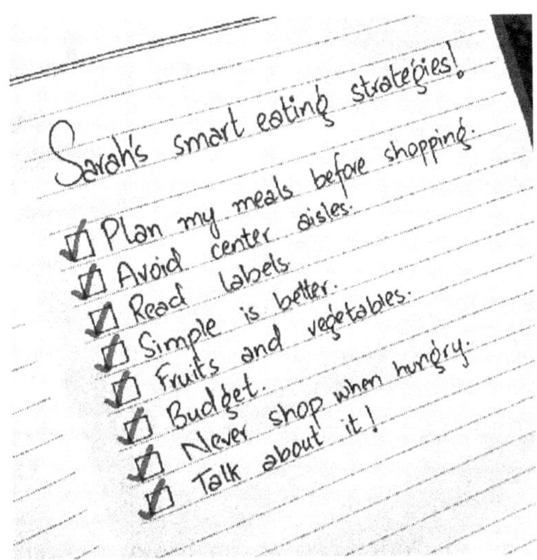

- ✓ Planning meals before shopping
- ✓ Avoid center aisles
- ✓ Read labels
- ✓ Simple is better
- ✓ Fruits and vegetables
- ✓ Budget
- ✓ Never shop when hungry
- ✓ Talk about it!

These was a good amount of investment in the form of time and energy in the making of this list. And these not only worked for Sarah, but these worked for me, for my friends and family, for Kyle from IT and even Karen from HR. If it can work for Karen, trust me, it can work for you too; Have a look.

Strategy # 1: *Shopping with intentions*

It's unbelievable how many people do not plan their meals before going to the store. I mean if you want to avoid the minefield of unhealthy choices, take a step back and plan your meals. Let me tell you how Sarah did it. The first step for her was to assess her needs and preferences. Ask yourself what are you trying to achieve. Losing weight, or simply healthy eating, whatever it is you have to figure it out and stick to it. Sarah always took a thorough look in her pantry and almost half the time she already had the majority of the ingredients required.

As Sarah went grocery shopping every week, she planned and mapped out her daily meals for the week. What she was going to have for breakfast, lunch, dinner and snacks. Her plan always included of a perfectly balanced and varied diet.

The next, and the most important thing she did was to write it all down. She made a habit of making a shopping list every time she had to go to the store and managed to save herself the frustration of coming home with a cart full of junk. You've got a plan, so follow it like your life depends on it. Because let's face it, your health does.

Strategy # 2: *Stay on track*

Sarah's second tactic, as soon as she entered the grocery store, was to shop at those areas of the store where fresh and unprocessed foods were predominately located. Usually these are at the perimeter of the store while the center aisles, like a maze, contains the processed food traps. If you want to avoid falling into the trap of unhealthy shopping, here's a pro tip: steer clear of the snack aisles. I know, I know, those brightly colored packages and tempting treats can be hard to resist, but trust me, it's for your own good.

Instead, fill up your cart with nutrient-dense goodies that will nourish your body and keep you satisfied. The hard part is to avoid those rows of chips and cookies. They are nothing but a one-way ticket to regret and guilt. The only way to avoid them is to stick firmly to the shopping list you have made. And if

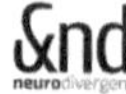

that doesn't work then adopt the "out of sight, out of mind" approach.

"But what if the products that I need *require* me to walk through the center aisles?" That's exactly the kind of thought that the mind of an addict would come up with. You could always ask one of the employees at the store to get you that particular 'healthy' product oh-so-conveniently placed in the middle of all processed food items. Come on, who are you trying to fool here?

Strategy # 3: *Ingredient investigation*

The next strategy that Sarah implemented was to use the power of reading labels. If she ever went in the processed food items aisles, she would pick up a product and flip it over to examine its ingredient list. Sarah always kept it simple. Take it this way; if she ever saw a laundry list of chemicals that she couldn't pronounce the product is going back to the shelf. If you think you need to know about each and every ingredient in that product, then focus on the eight categories of chemicals added in processed foods that I mentioned earlier in the previous chapter

Strategy # 4: *Uncomplicated choices*

This is more of a reminder than a strategy. Sarah had had enough of the complicated food nonsense. She was ready to ditch the convoluted ingredients in the fancy packaging. Sarah said goodbye to those mysterious chemicals and stuck with simple foods. You need to keep it real and keep it simple too. And it's time you showed those deceptive companies who's the boss of your health!

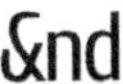

Strategy # 5: *Nature's multivitamins*

One of the ways Sarah avoided unhealthy shopping was to make a bold statement and hence she would fill her cart with fruits and vegetables – the real deal. I call them as nature's multivitamins. These products are powerhouses of nutrition because they are packed with minerals, vitamins, antioxidants and are our weapon against the onslaught of empty calories and artificial flavours. Once you fill up your cart with fruits and vegetables, you will have a sense of satisfaction which will make you realize that now purchasing unhealthy snacks is not just stupid but also a strain on your wallet.

Strategy # 6: *Wallet friendly wellness*

Budgeting is a tricky area. Sometimes when you are on a tight budget, you always have the option to choose convenience. It might not put out financial stress, but it can definitely compromise your health. In this case, always choose your health. But this is a rare scenario because majority of the convenient, processed junk is pretty expensive. Heck, the serving sizes alone rile me up! Most of these such items are heavy on the bank and choosing whole foods and unprocessed items is actually the best way to save both, your health, and your wealth.

A trick that Sarah implemented was to compare the company prices at various grocery stores. Sure, it will take some time for you to find the best and most cost-effective option, but once you do, you are going to save a lot of money. Just remember, budgeting isn't about the money anymore. It's a strategic weapon in the war against unhealthy shopping.

Strategy # 7: *Keep your cravings in check*

I want to have a chat with the snack enthusiast in you. Tell me, do you really want to get healthier and be able to make good

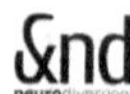

choices? Because if you don't have the will, there's no way for you, my friend. Close this book, get a packet of crisps, or chips, and have a movie marathon. On the other hand, if you have made up your mind to get rid of all those eating habits that are bad for your health, then I am about to help you with that.

The key is to not put yourself through a lot of restrain and limits, but to embrace the foodie in you. Let yourself choose freely. If you want to have a snack, go for something that is a healthier alternative and will still satisfy your tastebuds. For instance, when Sarah felt parched during summers and she just wanted to gulp down a whole bottle of juice kept in the fridge, she chose to have some watermelon. Juice was way easier but with just a little bit of an effort, she managed to save her health and satisfy her taste buds at the same time.

Flavourful fruits, crunchy vegetables, whole foods, all of these nourish your bodies and they do taste good. Just give them a chance and empty out your snack drawer. Get rid of your cookies and chips.

Strategy # 8: *Shop and connect*

Initially, when Sarah noticed how she would get easily tempted and buy unhealthy food products, she got scared that she might never be strong enough to bring such self-control to her. But luckily, Sarah was not alone. One day when she was in the gym, she recognized a familiar face. It was Iris, her downstairs neighbor. Iris had an introverted personality, or so Sarah had assumed, which is why she decided to say hi to Iris after the gym. Later when they both were making small talk, she found out that Iris goes to the same coffee shop where Sarah used to go. Sarah made a face when she heard about the coffee shop because after the truth about those granola bars were exposed, she had a tough time going back there. It was almost as if she was disappointed in that coffee shop instead of the

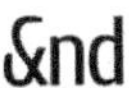

granola bar. Iris asked her about it, and she shared her journey. Turned out, Iris was just as health oriented as Sarah, and she found a potential companion in Iris. As time went by, they started spending a good amount of time together and because of their common preferences, they synchronized their timings for gym. Iris helped Sarah get comfortable in the coffee shop again, and Sarah accompanied her grocery shopping.

That was when Sarah noticed how she had started to avoid processed paraphernalia whenever she was with Iris. It might be due to the companionship and consideration for her friend, or it might be because Sarah was trying to subconsciously motivate healthy shopping to Iris. Either way, Sarah realized that she needed a good company with her in order to remain on the right track.

You need to seek out those like-minded individuals who understand not only you, but also the struggles you go through. Such shopping partners can offer motivation and encouragement. You also get to share your triumphs and tips and hold each other accountable. When those tempting aisles beckon, a supportive ally will be there to remind you of your goals and keep you on track. You need to think about who could accompany you to the market and help you maintain your healthy eating and healthy shopping habit. Once you do that, not only will you stay conscious of your choices, but your bank account will also thank you.

Just keep in mind that you are always the one in control of your thoughts. These strategies are just there to help you achieve your goals when it comes to healthy eating. But remember, the tips and tricks are not going to be your salvation, you are. These helping techniques are nothing but facilities for the long, full-of-struggle road trip to *Healthville*. Doesn't mean that they won't do you any good. Just give them a try and see for yourself.

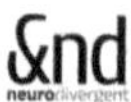

Part 2

Kitchen Alchemy 101: The Art of Guilt Free Indulgence

A playground for creativity; a gateway to a world where indulgence and health happily coexist is *kitchen alchemy*. This is an illuminating journey, and it will provoke you to rethink your approach to indulgence. Because of this, you will witness the magic when guilt-free diets, that defy the traditions, are created. Gone are the days of sacrificing taste for health. And no more settling for empty calories and remorseful binges. I will help you let go of the conventional ways using some simple food hacks and my personal favourite recipes. Fair warning for you, this could be considered as a rebellion against classic comfort foods. If you're okay with that, then you shall proceed. This is not your average cooking, my friend. It's an act of defiance against the norms of indulgence.

Food Hacks 101 – Culinary Shortcuts

The shortcuts and the clever techniques that not only make our life easier in the kitchen, but also enjoyable, are what I am calling *food hacks*. These are just like the little secrets that are whispered among food enthusiasts, specifically created to revolutionize the way people approach cooking, eating, and everything in between. So grab your apron and prepare to dive into the world of food hacks, where culinary creativity meets everyday convenience.

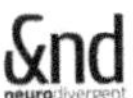

1. Prep and Conquer

In your extremely busy routine, skipping meals might be more frequent than you realize. I understand the hype and the busy life. I mean it is the 21st century and I am well aware of the dynamic routines that people have. Moreover, it gets really challenging when, amidst of the chaotic schedule, people face difficulty taking out some time to prepare and consume healthy meals. That is precisely when people like you orient towards processed meals unwillingly. Well, I've got the superhero of food hacks for you: meal prepping.

It not only saves time and effort, but it also helps you stay relaxed throughout your week because you don't have to stress out about eating and cooking healthy in a short amount of time. You must have seen those videos on the internet where people spend a few weekend hours chopping down vegetables, marinating proteins and pre-cooking grains. Well, get yourself some airtight containers, spend a few hours on the weekends and *voila*! You'll have a fridge stocked with ready-to-go ingredients. Now making meals will be a breeze when you're short on energy or time.

2. Gear Up Your Kitchen

Let's not underestimate the power of kitchen gadgets. These culinary instruments take your cooking game to a whole other level. Allow me to share some of my favorite kitchen gadgets that have saved a huge amount of time and effort.

- *Mandoline slicer:* I don't know where it got its name from, but this tool is used for the precise slicing and julienning of fruits and vegetables. These let you slice, chop, shred, dice and even all of these combined, depending upon the type you purchase. It totally eliminates the hassle of cutting a vegetable into slices of uniform thickness. You just have to take your food product, and run it through

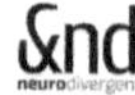

the blade of the slicer, and you will get a perfectly thin slice. The next time you swipe the vegetable onto the blade, it would cut another slice of the same thickness. Some of these slicers even have knobs for you to adjust the thickness. Just a tip, whenever you are slicing any food product, lets say a cucumber, just make sure that when you reach to the base, use the palm of your hand instead of your fingers to slice the rest of the vegetable. That way you can ensure the safety of your hand. After using this device, you have thin beautiful slices of your vegetable in just a matter of seconds. And I'm not even exaggerating!

- *Multiblade herb scissors:* I recently got my hands on this one and trust me when I say that the person who came up with these is a genius! I always had a hard time chopping down some fresh coriander just because the leaves would fly out all over the place. This just reduced my meal prep time in half because not only can I cut coriander leaves using this gadget, but I can also cut tomatoes, cucumbers, and many other such herbs.

- *Salad spinner:* I have some really good, tried-and-tested recipes for various kinds of salads – which I will be sharing with you in a while, don't worry – but the problem I used to face while making a salad bowl was the moisture content. Laurel from Marketing once saw me Google this issue on my computer and suggested me a salad spinner. As much as I felt like she invaded my personal space, she was also right.

Not only did my salad spinner dried down the freshly cut and rinsed vegetables, it is also now being used as a part of my meal prepping procedures. On weekends I take some time to clean out the vegetables and put them in the storage compartments in the fridge. But not before using this device and making sure that the maximum

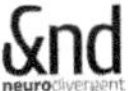

moisture has been spun out of the product just to avoid microbial attack. This way I don't have to go through the process of washing, rinsing and drying my vegetables whenever I want to make any meal. So convenient!

- *Garlic press:* This is the one gadget that you might not realize you need unless you actually use it. Using a grater to get garlic to be minced or finely chopped is old school and isn't exactly convenient. With one forceful push, you get a whole clove of garlic finely chopped. These are very easy to wash and oh, one more thing, you can use this for many other vegetables, like small portions of onions, ginger, olives etc. The possibilities are endless.

- *Spiralizer:* This is one of my favorite kitchen tools and it is used to create vegetable noodles, for instance zucchini noodles. You simply have to place the vegetable you want to spiralize, let's say zucchini, and once it's fixed in the gadget, you start rotating the knob and out comes spiralized zucchini. As simple as it sounds. Some spiralizers come with various blades that can be fixed, and taken out, for a different shape and / or thickness of the vegetable noodle. One of my favorite blades is the straight one, that makes these beautiful cucumber ribbons that instantly make my salad look gourmet. Speaking of zucchini noodles, I'll definitely share this delicious recipe soon.

- *Air fryer:* Air fryers might not be the most economy-friendly gadget, but they solve one of the major health issues when it comes to eating fried food – the oil. Actually, you know what, I change my statement. Air fryers are economy-friendly when it comes to the bills. These are more cost effective than the ovens we normally use. Not only can you use an air fryer for snacks like homemade nuggets or healthy chips, but you can also use this for vegetables, like broccoli, zucchini, mushrooms and

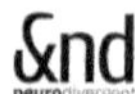

onions. Moreover, it works just as well with proteins like chicken drumsticks, pork, meatballs, tofu, etc. Now you can enjoy your favorite snack and still maintain a healthy nutritional balance.

There are so many other useful gadgets as well, for instance the egg separator or the silicon baking mats, but the ones I have mentioned are specifically designed to reduce time consumption and effort. These are a holy grail for people like you.

3. DIY Chips

I know your mind must be hovering around the homemade chips I mentioned just now. Well this is one of my most favorite and most used hack ever. I have always loved the salty – savory flavor bursts that comes with these processed chips and crisps but boy are these bad for you. Due to countless hours of research on healthy eating, I came across this article by *thespruceeats* on making my own chips. And not just using potatoes only, but using so many different vegetables like kale, zucchini, butternut squash, sweet potato, beets, carrots, parsnips, even the vegetable peels! So many options had me excited for healthy snacking. Just use a Mandoline slicer, cut thin slices of the vegetable, add seasoning and put them in an oven to bake, or in an air fryer. Either way you will get a much healthier and better alternative to the processed and packaged potato chips you get from the store. Keep an eye out for the recipes for these.

4. Frozen Temptations

One thing that always took most of my effort to get over was ice cream. When I found out that ice creams not only have added sugars, but also saturated fats, I was devastated and felt like this healthy eating practice is not worth it. I

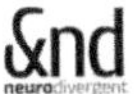

tried to keep myself away from ice cream, but I was like an addict! Until one night, my ice cream cravings had me make mango milkshake and keep it in the freezer. I was eager to see if my homemade ice cream would come out just as delicious as the ones I crave or not. Heck, I was even expecting a better taste. Turned out, it tasted horrible. The milkshake froze completely, making it impossible for me to drink it so I waited for it to defrost. And when it did, it was really unpleasant, to say the least. I didn't know where and how things went wrong but I refused to give up. Finally, with some help from the internet, I figured out an easy hack to make homemade ice creams: freeze some ripe fruits first, like bananas, and then blend them into a creamy, guilt-free treat. With a little determination and some clever ingredient substitutions, I managed to satisfy my cravings without derailing my healthy eating goals. How cool is that? Pun intended.

5. Taste Upgrade

Salt and pepper might be the dynamic duo of kitchen but why stop there? Try elevating and upgrading your dish with a sprinkle of smoked paprika, a dash of cayenne pepper, or a squeeze of fresh lemon juice; some of my favorite flavor enhancements. Embrace the audacity to experiment with natural sweeteners like maple syrup and dates. Try experimenting with herbs, spices, and citrus foods to awaken your taste buds and transform even the simplest meals into culinary masterpieces.

6. Leftover Makeover

Giving your leftover meals a second chance is what kitchen alchemy is all about! For instance, once I wanted to make myself a sandwich for breakfast. Having every ingredient in

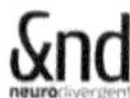

my fridge, it was no problem for me to fix up one quickly. I had the bread, the vegetables, and some boneless chicken cubes in the freezer as well. When I assembled it all, I took out the chicken cubes and thought on how to season and marinate it. 'If I could just mimic the flavor from the roasted chicken I had last night,' is what I thought. And that was when realization hit me, and I took out the leftover chicken from the fridge. After shredding it and incorporating it into the sandwich, I tasted it. And believe me when I say this, that it was the best sandwich I had ever made.

It's not just sandwiches though, I have used such leftover chicken for making salads. I have also utilized leftover rice by mixing it with some sauces and sautéed vegetables (recipe coming to you soon). Don't let those leftovers go to waste. Instead, let them inspire you to create something new and exciting.

7. Hack Attack

Apart from food hacks, let me share some of the most common and useful kitchen hacks that are going to reduce your meal prepping time and make your kitchen life so much easier. These small but mighty hacks will save you from kitchen disasters and keep your meals on track. Get ready for a hack attack:

- Use a cheese grater to easily grate solid butter or cooking chocolate for baking recipes. You might want to let the chocolate get a little soft for efficient and quick grating.
- Freeze leftover coffee in an ice cube tray to use for iced coffee without diluting the flavor.
- Put a damp paper towel under a cutting board to keep it from slipping while you chop.
- Sprinkle salt on a cutting board before slicing garlic to prevent it from sticking to the knife.

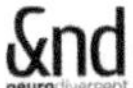

- Store leftover herbs in an ice cube tray with olive oil for convenient and flavorful additions to your dishes.
- Use a muffin tin to bake individual portions of mac and cheese for perfectly portioned servings.
- Microwave a lemon for a few seconds before squeezing to extract more juice.
- Running your knife under hot water makes slicing through sticky foods smooth like butter.
- Place a wooden spoon over a boiling pot prevents it from bubbling over
- Freeze leftover wine in ice cube trays to add to sauces or stews for an instant flavor boost.
- Dip cookie cutters in flour before using them to prevent the dough from sticking.
- Rub stainless steel on your hands to remove strong odors like garlic or onion.
- Wrap the stems of bananas with plastic wrap to keep them fresh longer.
- Use dental floss to effortlessly slice through soft foods like cheese or cake layers.

I could go on and on about these kitchen hacks, but you get the idea, right? This is how mealtime has always been a success for me. Try some of these hacks and conquer the kitchen with your newfound knowledge.

Now is the time for you to revolutionize your kitchen. With a hint of sass and a dash of attitude, you can easily turn your guilty pleasures into guilt-free triumphs. Now tell me, are you going to take a stand against mediocrity, and dare to be different?

"Sure, but Muneeba, what about those recipes?" Relax, I am a man of my words. Besides, good things come to those who wait. Fortunately for you, the wait is over. Let us begin with the recipe revolution.

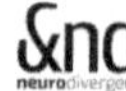

Flavor Fusion 101 – From Meals to Masterpieces

So you're looking for easy recipes, huh? Well, lucky for you, I'm here to rescue you from your culinary incompetence. Simple recipes, for those who struggle to boil water without burning it. Yes, even you, the master of kitchen disasters, can attempt these foolproof creations. Okay, picture this: a basic omelet, because cracking an egg is about the extent of your culinary prowess. Toss in some random veggies you found in the fridge, hope they're not rotten, and sprinkle some cheese on top. Does that sound to complicated? My dear inept cook, put on your ill-fitting apron and attempt these simple recipes. Let's begin with my most favorite one ever:

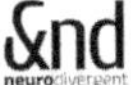

Salad Symphony

Salads are the epitome of freshness, flavor and health. Now since it is not a recipe book, I'm only going to share my favorite ones here. So, without further ado, let's dive into a world of vibrant colors, crisp textures, and tantalizing tastes with these mouthwatering salad recipes.

1. Taco Salad

Try something new for once. Explore the flavors beyond the realm of tacos and get creative with salads. Here's what you need to do:

Ingredients:

- ✓ 4 Tortilla Taco
- ✓ 1 lb. lean ground beef
- ✓ 3 Tbsp Taco Seasoning
- ✓ 1/2 cup water
- ✓ 1 iceberg lettuce, chopped
- ✓ 1 avocado, sliced
- ✓ 1/2 cup tortilla strips or chips
- ✓ 1/4 cup cilantro, chopped
- ✓ 1 lime which is optional

Steps:

- ✓ Cook your beef in a large skillet and spoon out all the excess fat.

- ✓ Add in taco seasoning and water, and cook for 3 – 5 minutes, stirring occasionally.

- ✓ Remove from heat and cool.

Nutrition Facts	
Servings 4	
Amount per serving	
Calories	569
	% Daily Value*
Total Fat 41g	63%
Saturated Fat 12g	75%
Cholesterol 105 mg	35%
Sodium 885 mg	38%
Total Carbohydrates 25g	8%
Dietary Fiber 6g	25%
Total sugars 9g	
Protein 30g	
Vitamin C 21 mg	25%
Vitamin A 1470IU	29%
Calcium 187 mg	19%
Iron 4 mg	22%

**The % Daily Value (DV) tells you how much a nutrient in a food serving contributes to a daily diet. 2,000 calories a day is used for general nutrition advice.*

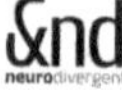

✓ Add your desired dressing and stir to combine. Refrigerate it.

✓ Prepare your toppings and add them along with a cilantro garnish.

✓ Squeeze some lime and serve.

Salads have always been the easiest and rawest of the recipes. You're literally just combining raw, unprocessed food into a delicious mixture. Let me share one more recipe with you.

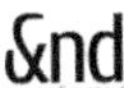

2. Macaroni Salad

Macaroni salad is the perfect side dish for a barbeque, or burgers. Here's how to make it:

Ingredients for salad:

✓ 2 cups elbow macaroni, cooked according to package instructions
✓ 1 cup diced red bell peppers
✓ 1/2 cup diced red onion
✓ 1/2 cup diced celery
✓ 2 hard-boiled eggs
✓ 1 Tbsp chopped parsley for garnishing

Ingredients for dressing:

✓ 1/2 cup mayonnaise
✓ 3 tbsp apple cider vinegar
✓ 3 tsp yellow mustard
✓ 1 tsp black pepper, ground
✓ 1 tsp salt

Steps:

✓ Gather all the ingredients for dressing and combine them in a bowl. Whisk until smooth and creamy.

✓ Place the cooked macaroni in a bowl, along with the ingredients for the salad.

✓ Combine the salad mixture and the dressing mixture together and garnish with fresh parsley leaves.

✓ Refrigerate, and serve.

Nutrition Facts	
Servings 6	
Amount per serving	
Calories	348
	% Daily Value*
Total Fat 16g	25%
Saturated Fat 3g	19%
Cholesterol 62 mg	21%
Sodium 627 mg	27%
Total Carbohydrates 41g	14%
Dietary Fiber 3g	13%
Total sugars 5g	
Protein 9g	
Vitamin C 33 mg	40%
Vitamin A 1002IU	20%
Calcium 32 mg	3%
Iron 1 mg	6%

*The % Daily Value (DV) tells you how much a nutrient in a food serving contributes to a daily diet. 2,000 calories a day is used for general nutrition advice.

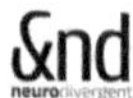

The classic macaroni salad is by far one of the tastiest salads you'll ever have.

Whether you crave something light and refreshing, or a proper meal in a bowl, these salad recipes will satisfy your taste buds and nourish your body at the same time. There was such variety of recipes, from tuna salad to a brussels sprout salad, but that's for you to discover by embarking on a culinary adventure filled with bold flavors and endless possibilities.

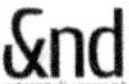

DIY Crispy Crunches

We all know how chips have always had a special place in our hearts (and taste buds), but they aren't exactly the poster child for health. Well, get ready to have your mind blown because these chip recipes are about to shatter your snacking expectations!

1. Baked potato-chips:

The first on is super simple. Before you start, make sure you have sliced your potato. For that you may use a mandolin slicer. Once you have your slices ready, here is what you'll need to do.

Ingredients:

- ✓ 1 potato, sliced
- ✓ 1 tablespoon olive oil
- ✓ 1/4 teaspoon salt

Steps:

- ✓ Gather all the ingredients.

- ✓ Preheat the oven at temperature 450 F. I usually coat my baking sheet with a cooking spray.

- ✓ Toss those freshly cut potato slices in a bowl with olive oil and salt.

- ✓ Place the potato slices on the baking sheet, make sure no piece overlaps the other.

- ✓ Put the tray in the oven and bake for about 10 to 12 minutes. If the chips

Nutrition Facts

Servings 4

Amount per serving	
Calories	140

	% Daily Value*
Total Fat 4g	5%
Saturated Fat 1g	3%
Cholesterol 0 mg	0%
Sodium 148 mg	6%
Total Carbohydrates 24g	9%
Dietary Fiber 3g	9%
Total sugars 1g	
Protein 3g	

Vitamin C 9 mg	47%
Calcium 21 mg	2%
Iron 1 mg	7%
Potassium 624 mg	13%

The % Daily Value (DV) tells you how much a nutrient in a food serving contributes to a daily diet. 2,000 calories a day is used for general nutrition advice.

become light golden in color before 10 minutes, then you may take them out. Just make sure that they don't turn brown, which would mean that the potato slice is overcooked.

✓ After they've cooled down, you may serve and enjoy.

Also, if you add in some *barbeque seasoning*, you got your own homemade healthy barbecue chips! Prepare to take your health game to the next level with a mouthwatering suggestion: dive into the world of homemade barbecue seasoning recipe. Here's the one I use:

✓ Paprika 1/2 cup
✓ Fine kosher salt 1/4 cup
✓ Granulated sugar 1/4 cup
✓ Mustard powder 2 tablespoons
✓ Chili powder 1/4 cup
✓ Ground cumin 1/4 cup
✓ Black pepper (freshly ground) 2 tablespoons
✓ Garlic 1/4 cup
✓ Cayenne 2 tablespoons.

Mix all these in a jar and you have your own barbeque seasoning! Instead of deep frying, when you bake the chips, you will be lowering the fat intake while still being able to enjoy a crispy crunchy snack.

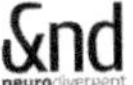

2. Vegetable chips:

So you think potatoes are the only vegetable that can be made into chips? Think again. Making homemade vegetable chips is extremely easy, doesn't matter whether you fry them or you bake them. Moreover, making your own veggie chips is exciting because you get to choose the vegetable. Let me share my thoughts and choices on this one. For me, root vegetables are my number one choice, like potatoes, beets, carrots, parsnips etc. Allow me to share with you how these vegetable chips are made:

Ingredients:

- ✓ 1 large carrot
- ✓ 1 large parsnip
- ✓ 1 sweet potato
- ✓ 1 large beet
- ✓ Canola oil

Seasoning mix:

- ✓ 2 teaspoons kosher salt
- ✓ 1/4 teaspoon garlic powder
- ✓ 1/4 teaspoon onion powder

Make sure the vegetables are peeled and thinly sliced before you begin

Steps:

- ✓ Gather all the ingredients and heat the oil (for frying) upto 350 F.

- ✓ Take a bowl and fill it with ice water.

- ✓ Add the thin slices of the carrot, parsnip and potato into the bowl

Nutrition Facts	
Servings 6	
Amount per serving	
Calories	313
	% Daily Value*
Total Fat 25g	32%
Saturated Fat 2g	9%
Cholesterol 0 mg	0%
Sodium 456 mg	20%
Total Carbohydrates 23g	8%
Dietary Fiber 4g	15%
Total sugars 5g	
Protein 2g	
Vitamin C 13 mg	67%
Calcium 33 mg	3%
Iron 1 mg	6%
Potassium 555 mg	12%

**The % Daily Value (DV) tells you how much a nutrient in a food serving contributes to a daily diet. 2,000 calories a day is used for general nutrition advice.*

✓ Add the beet slices in a separate bowl of ice water

✓ Let the vegetables sit for about 30 minutes

✓ Drain out the vegetable slices and place them in the heated oil.

✓ Fry them until they appear golden brown and crisp.

✓ Place them on a paper towel and once slightly less hot, add in the seasoning mix and toss the chips around to coat them evenly with the seasoning.

✓ Serve and enjoy.

You can store these chips in an airtight jar for up to two days. Moreover, this recipe is not just limited to vegetables, you can make such crispy snacks using fruits and vegetable peels as well. Of course you would have to wash clean and dry the peels prior, and you can also bake them instead of frying. How amazing is that!

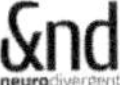

Baked tortilla chips:

Not only dos this recipe satisfy my savory cravings, but it also is a lot less messy to create. With baked tortilla chips you definitely need a homemade salsa recipe, obviously. Here's how I make the salsa:

Ingredients:

- ✓ 2 cups finely chopped tomatoes
- ✓ 2 cloves garlic, pressed or minced
- ✓ 1/4 teaspoon sea salt
- ✓ 1 tablespoon lime juice
- ✓ 2 tablespoons minced fresh cilantro
- ✓ 1 tablespoon minced red onion
- ✓ 1/2 teaspoon ground cumin
- ✓ 1/2 teaspoon chili powder
- ✓ 1/4 teaspoon cayenne pepper
- ✓ 1 teaspoon minced and chili pepper, for example jalapeño pepper

Steps:

- ✓ Gather the ingredients

- ✓ Mix tomatoes, garlic, salt and lime in a bowl.

- ✓ Now incorporate other optional ingredients like onion, jalapeño, cayenne, cumin etc.

- ✓ Mix gently and refrigerate, until ready to serve.

Now that your homemade salsa is ready, let's move on to the main recipe, tortilla chips:

Nutrition Facts	
Servings 4	
Amount per serving	
Calories	53
	% Daily Value*
Total Fat 1g	1%
Saturated Fat 0g	1%
Cholesterol 0 mg	0%
Sodium 81 mg	4%
Total Carbohydrates 11g	4%
Dietary Fiber 2g	5%
Total sugars 0g	
Protein 1g	
Vitamin C 0 mg	0%
Calcium 19 mg	1%
Iron 0 mg	2%
Potassium 45 mg	1%

The % Daily Value (DV) tells you how much a nutrient in a food serving contributes to a daily diet. 2,000 calories a day is used for general nutrition advice.

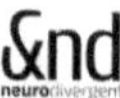

Ingredients:
- ✓ Corn tortillas
- ✓ Cooking spray
- ✓ Butter
- ✓ 1/8 teaspoon salt

Steps:

- ✓ Gather all the ingredients and preheat the oven upto 200 F.

- ✓ Take the 4 tortillas and place them on top of each other.

- ✓ Now cut them in half, and again cut them in quarters, and again cut inti further triangles making a total of 8 tortilla triangles per piece.

- ✓ Grease the baking sheet with butter, or better yet, use a cooking spray that's butter flavored, and place the tortilla triangles onto the tray.

- ✓ Sprinkle salt over them, and place the tortilla triangles into the oven, baking them for 10 minutes.

- ✓ Take them out until they become crisp, or another indication is when their corners start to go brown.

- ✓ Serve with homemade salsa and enjoy.

It is safe to say that this is one of my most favorite homemade chips recipe and the way it makes my tastebuds explode with pleasure, is something that can only be understood with experience. So go on and try this one right now.

These healthy chips are low in calories but high in flavor, so you can satisfy your snack cravings without compromising your health goals. So the next time your snack radar goes off, reach for one of these game-changing chip recipes and let your taste buds dance with delight. Trust us, your snacking hour just got a whole lot exciting!

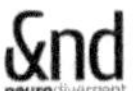

Frozen Fantasies

Getting to know that I can indulge in my favorite comfort food, without the unhealthy effects, was like a dream. I came to know about some chemical substances that are added in ice creams and what makes them unhealthy. For instance, carrageenan, cellulose gum, artificial colors, partially hydrogenated oils, artificial colors, soybean oil etc. healthy ice creams are the ones that require minimum ingredients. Let me share some of the most enticing flavors of homemade ice cream with you.

1. Vanilla ice cream

This vanilla ice cream recipe has only 4 ingredients. It includes a natural sweetener like maple syrup, so it is a bonus that artificial sugars have been avoided. Here's what you'll need to do:

Nutrition Facts	
Servings 5 cups	
Amount per serving (0.5 cups)	
Calories	90
	% Daily Value*
Total Fat 1g	2%
Saturated Fat 1g	5%
Potassium 48 mg	1%
Sodium 2 mg	0%
Total Carbohydrates 15g	5%
Dietary Fiber 1g	4%
Total sugars 14g	
Protein 1g	
Calcium 33 mg	3%

The % Daily Value (DV) tells you how much a nutrient in a food serving contributes to a daily diet. 2,000 calories a day is used for general nutrition advice.

Ingredients:

✓ 3 1/3 cups full fat coconut milk

✓ 1/2 cup regular unsweetened milk of choice like almond milk

✓ 1/3 cup maple syrup

✓ 2 tsp vanilla extract

Steps:

Follow these steps if you have an ice cream maker:

✓ Add all the ingredients in a large mixing bowl.

✓ Stir them and transfer the mixture to the ice cream maker.

✓ Follow the instructions according to the ice cream maker you are using.

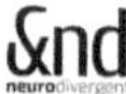

✓ Once done, freeze for 3 - 4 hours and serve.

What if you don't have an ice cream maker? Follow these steps:

✓ Add all the ingredients in a large mixing bowl.

✓ Stir them and transfer the mixture to a zip lock bag.

✓ Place the bag in the freezer for about 3 hours.

✓ Take out the frozen mixture and blend it. You can add cream or milk, according to your preference..

✓ Put it again in the freezer for at least 3 – 4 hours, or overnight.

You can see for yourself from this recipe that this ice cream is made from clean and healthy ingredients. Look at the coconut milk; it has fiber, proteins, and minerals like magnesium, potassium, iron etc. This is a definite upgrade from the store-bought ice creams. Anyway, let's move on to other flavors.

Other flavors you might not want to miss:

Now that you know how to make vanilla ice cream, here are some other fun flavors that you can enjoy. The method of preparation is the same for each.

✓ *Choco-Banana ice cream*: Add 3 bananas, 1/4 tsp pure vanilla extract, a pinch of salt, and 3 tbsp cocoa powder.

✓ *Mint Choco Chip:* Add 2 bananas, a pinch of salt, 1/8 tsp peppermint extract, and stir in chocolate chips blending.

✓ *Piña Colada:* Add 1/4 cup coconut milk, 1/2 cup frozen pineapple. You may also add shredded coconut.

With these recipes, I've managed to make my frozen fantasies into a reality. And you know what the best part is? They don't even require much effort.

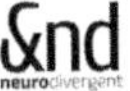

Sensational Sauté

A vegetable stir fry is always a delicious addition to a meal, like rice, noodles, steak or stuffed chicken. This one-pan dish can also be served as a main course on its own.

Ingredients:

- ✓ 1 sliced carrot
- ✓ 2 cups broccoli
- ✓ 8 oz can of baby corn
- ✓ 8 oz sliced mushrooms
- ✓ 1 whole sliced pepper
- ✓ 2 Tbsp cooking oil
- ✓ 2 Tbsp unsalted butter
- ✓ 3 minced garlic cloves
- ✓ 2 tsp minced ginger

Steps:

- ✓ Heat the oil, and add all the vegetables, stirring for about 3 minutes until the vegetables are crisp and tender at the same time. Yeah, that's a thing, crisp-tender.

- ✓ Add butter, ginger and garlic and cook until you feel its fragrance.

- ✓ And add any sauce of your choice, and stir fry for 3 – 4 minutes until the sauce thickens, and serve

Nutrition Facts	
Servings 4	
Amount per serving	
Calories	256
	% Daily Value*
Total Fat 5g	22%
Saturated Fat 5g	31%
Potassium 603 mg	17%
Sodium 444 mg	19%
Total Carbohydrates 31g	10%
Dietary Fiber 4g	17%
Total sugars 15g	
Protein 7g	
Vitamin A 4089IU	82%
Vitamin C 85 mg	103%
Calcium 30 mg	3%
Iron 1 mg	6%

**The % Daily Value (DV) tells you how much a nutrient in a food serving contributes to a daily diet. 2,000 calories a day is used for general nutrition advice.*

So, there you have it. These 'oh-so-complicated' recipes might just help you stumble your way through meal prepping and even cooking. They may not earn you a Michelin star, but at least you'll avoid setting your kitchen on fire.

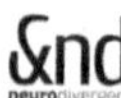

If you haven't figured it out yet, meal planning, grocery shopping and cooking are essential skills you should have mastered by now. Seriously, get it together. If you need a push, a head start, allow me: start by actually taking the time to create a weekly meal plan. It's not rocket science. And when you make your grocery list, please, for the love of all, stick to it. I mean, think about it, is it really that hard to resist those tempting, impulse buys? Moreover, stick to the perimeter of the store, where the healthy stuff is usually located. I shouldn't have to tell you that because we've already talked about it. And while you're at it, why not consider using seasonal ingredients? They're cheaper and taste better. It's not like it requires a PhD in culinary arts to figure that out. Now, when it comes to cooking, how about you try batch cooking? It's a concept that's been around for ages. You cook a bunch of food at once and *voilà*, you have leftovers! But hey, if you can't be bothered, at least invest in some fancy kitchen gadgets which might save you from burning down the kitchen. Just remember, kitchen alchemy is your battleground, and guilt-free indulgence is your ultimate triumph.

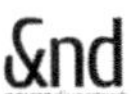

CHAPTER
4

Food for Thought – Our Nutritional Compass

Here's one thing that I can never understand: why is it so hard for you to grasp the importance of incorporating evidence-based recommendations for healthy eating? Everyone knows how our choices have a direct impact on our bodies and overall wellbeing, both physically and mentally. And yet, instead of relying on sound advice backed by evidence, you continue to fall for fad diets and misinformation. Is it rocket science?

To answer my question for you, no it is not rocket science, my friend. Nutrient-rich, whole foods should always be the foundation of your diet because you need those essential vitamins, minerals, and antioxidants. But what do you do? You reach for processed junk filled with artificial additives, unhealthy fats, and excessive amounts of salt. And then you wonder why you are at a higher risk of obesity, heart disease, and other chronic conditions.

And don't even get me started on portion control. It feels like common sense has gone down the drain, and out the window. People like you stuff themselves with oversized portions, which eventually leads to weight gain and a whole lot of health problems. Instead, you should just listen to your body and eat only until you're satisfied. Moderation is key, always remember that.

What's more is that, instead of drinking an adequate amount of water each day, you choose to walk around in a dehydrated haze wondering why you feel fatigued, and why your skin looks dull. Maybe if you had paid attention to your basic bodily needs,

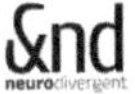

you'd realize the importance of staying properly hydrated. And those cooking methods? Boy, do those get on my nerves! It's incomprehensible how people like you can think that deep-frying everything you can get their hands on is a healthy choice. Hello? Do you not realize that frying adds unnecessary fats and calories to your already poor food choices? You should just put in a little effort to steam, boil, grill, or bake your food. This way you could actually hold on to some nutritional value.

Don't pout now, you're making me feel bad for giving you a reality check.

"Let's back it up by science!"

The evidence that I am talking about is about to be presented in front of you. Allow me to simplify things for you and put up a list of the evidence-based recommendations. Have a look.

- Focusing on whole foods
- Moderation is the key
- Practice mindful eating
- Limit added sugars
- Reduce sodium intake
- Individualize your diet

From Farm to Fork

You must be going, 'here we go again with the whole "eat your fruits and vegetables" thing', like you haven't heard that a million times before, but I can't emphasize enough how unprocessed foods are a fundamental cornerstone of optimal nutrition. Choosing unprocessed foods is a conscious decision where you prioritize quality and nourishment. In a nutshell, here's why they're essential:

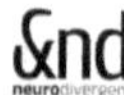

Fruits and vegetables offer a plethora of vitamins, minerals, and phytochemicals that contribute to our vitality. Whole grains, in their natural form, provide valuable fiber and other important nutrients that often are lost in refined forms. Lean proteins offer essential amino acids that your body needs for growth, repair, and overall proper functioning. Healthy fats provide essential fatty acids that are actually good for the health.

The question here is, how to focus on whole foods. Here are a few tips and tricks for you:

- The easiest way to focus on something is preparation. Try planning out your meals and make sure your mind revolves around the healthy eating strategies. A part of *planning and preparation* is to make a list of the ingredients that you need. This will help you focus on the unprocessed ingredients only.
- You can also try the *'out of sight, out of mind'* approach and stay in those areas of the grocery stores that contain whole, unprocessed foods. It works wonders, trust me.
- Labels are a big help for you. Pick up a product and read its label. If it contain the *minimum amount of ingredients* and nothing 'artificial' in it, you can definitely go for it. Otherwise put that product back and just leave the aisle.
- Another trick to make sure that out diet consists of unprocessed, whole foods, is to keep your *fridge stocked up on fruits and vegetables*. That way you can always go for healthy snacking and incorporate into meals or smoothies. You can also snack on a handful of nuts. The possibilities are endless.
- Do make sure about your *protein source*, because poultry, fish, legumes, tofu, Greek yogurt are a few examples of lean proteins. These are much more nutritious and will satisfy you for much longer.

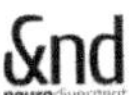

- One way to keep your mind focused on consuming whole foods is to get excited about it. Search for new recipes and *have fun experimenting with cooking*. Roasting, grilling and steaming are some great techniques to enhance the natural flavors of whole foods.

Just keep in mind that choosing unprocessed, whole foods is not a deprivation, it is an upgrade. You aren't sacrificing taste, instead you're embracing the abundance of flavors and textures that nature provides.

The Goldilocks Approach

You remember Goldilocks? She had to choose between two extremes and opted for the perfect and the balanced option. In the realm of healthy diet and nutrition, the Goldilocks approach is when you find the ideal solution that lies between two opposite ends of a spectrum, where neither extreme is desirable. It is also about finding a balanced diet that includes a variety of nutrient-dense foods without being overly restrictive or indulgent. It encourages moderation and portion control, rather than excessive or insufficient consumption and here's how you can achieve said moderation:

- *Controlling your portions* and being mindful of your portion sizes. You can use smaller lates and bowls if you don't have that kind of self-control yet. This will help create an illusion of a fuller plate. And do not limit your portion to 1 food group, instead, add in proteins, carbohydrates, vegetables and grains.
- To maintain moderation, you have got to *listen to your body*. Learn to distinguish between your physical hunger, and your mindless and emotional binge-eating. Before you reach for a snack, take a pause and ask yourself, are you really hungry? It is possible that you might have

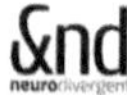

reached out for that snack just for comfort and / or distraction.

- One important thing to keep in mind is to realize that *moderation is not deprivation*. Allow yourself to indulge in your favorite treats, while keeping a check and balance.
- If you feel like you may have an eating disorder, which does not allow you to maintain a balance, you need to get *professional and medical help*. There is absolutely nothing to worry about if you have been diagnosed, and all that professional help would do, is provide guidance and help you develop a healthy relationship with food.

Moderation is always the key. And this balance will not only help you with your food related issues, but also in many other aspects of life. But for now, start with your diet, make thoughtful decisions and always consider the potential consequences of extremes.

Mindful Eating

The fact that I have to explain this is already starting to aggravate me. Mindful eating is not some groundbreaking concept that requires a degree in rocket science. It's about paying attention to what you are putting in your mouth. It's about savoring every bite, every moment of your meal instead of inhaling it like a ravenous animal. Our distractions like televisions and mobile phones are the number one enemies of mindful eating.

Now I am going to share some strategies with you that have been scientifically proven to determine that mindful eating is possibly an effective tool against unfavorable eating behaviors like binge eating, and emotional eating, which eventually leads up to obesity, weight gain and other health issues. Here are seven research-based strategies on how to achieve mindful eating:

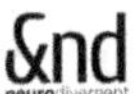

1. *Honor and acknowledge the food.* Think about who prepared it, where did the ingredients come from, how was it prepared. This will immediately deepen your relationship with your food.
2. *Use all your senses.* Observe the colors, textures, scents and fragrances, tastes and the mouthfeel of the food on your plate.
3. *Modest proportions* are going to allow you to value your food. Do not add in excess. A trick is to use a smaller dinner plate and fill it up only once. Not only will this avoid overeating but will also avoid food being wasted.
4. *Slowing down* is one of the was to savor your meal. Take small bites and do not swallow it after chewing for a few rimes. In fact, you need to chew your food thoroughly so that it can initiate digestion.
5. When a *meal is skipped*, I increases the risk of strong feelings of hunger, and that can lead to the easiest and quickest food choices, which are majority of the time, not healthy. Such risks are reduced when you plan and fix a time for your meals.
6. Always *avoid distractions* during your mealtime. Turn off the TV, Put away your phone and create a calm and peaceful environment for yourself.
7. *Practice gratitude* once you're given the meal, as it is a blessing to have food on your plate, once you're eating it, as it tastes good and is going to be the energy you later utilize, and once after the meal, on how it makes you feel satisfied and ready for your next task.

A review of literature of 68 observational studies found out that slowing down the speed of a meal allows us to recognize the feeling of fullness. Mindful eating provides sufficient time for our bodies to determine when the food intake should be stopped, hence, makes you have a greater control over it.

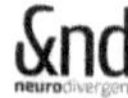

Now, tell me something, did you really needed to be told about mindful eating? Was it all necessary that I lecture you like all our moms to sit down at the table, put away your phones and actually taste the food?

Sweet Surrender

It seems like apparently you need to be reminded over and over again to avoid sugars. I guess it could mean that you are stubborn, or maybe you need some help to give this food group up. Here are some tips for you to avoid sugar substances.

- Always read the *food labels* to check the ingredient list. Look for any added sugars, or artificial sweeteners. Terms like sucrose, fructose, glucose, corn syrup etc., are the ones you need to look out for.
- *Whole foods* are naturally low in sugar, so these are the perfect ingredients for your recipe.
- If you can't resist sweetness, you can add in *natural sweeteners* yourself like fruits, or maple syrup, or honey, or even vanilla extract. These alternatives can enhance the flavor without relying on refined sugars.
- Always *avoid the low-fat* or fat-free foods because when fats are removed, the companies compensate for the loss of flavor by adding in artificial sweeteners.
- To *satisfy your sweet tooth*, you can definitely make some treats at home. Like ice creams. Instead of relying on store bought desserts, try making your own sweet snack at home. You have control over the ingredients and can choose healthier alternat.
- *Drink water* instead of sugary beverages and sodas. I know you order a fizzy drink with your meals when you're dining out. But for once, try and have your meal with water only.

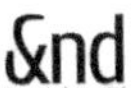

You know, sometimes I can't believe that we're still having such conversations about sugars. How many times do you need to hear that sugar is the devil? It feels like you all are a bunch of children who can't control your own cravings. Newsflash, you all are adults, capable of making your own choices.

Shake the Salt

Alright my salty companion, you know excessive sodium intake can harm your body. I mean, I really get it, the flavor is important. But do you really need to drown everything in a sea of salt? To be honest, our taste buds deserve more than just an explosive one-dimensional bomb of sodium. You'll be amazed at how much better food tastes when you're not constantly reaching for the saltshaker. Here are some tips and tricks to help you reduce salt intake:

- *Cook from scratch*. By doing this you have a better control of the sodium proportion that goes in the meal. Instead of relying on salt for taste, use herbs and spices to give a burst of flavors.
- *Rinsing the canned food* products is one trick that I saw others doing and yet had no idea what was happening. Until recently when I was in my kitchen, preparing a quick meal, I rinsed some canned beans, with the intention to remove some of the saltiness as I had had an unpleasant experience previously, and I instantly realized that this was why people did it.
- *Go easy on the condiments*. The spices and ingredients added in processed condiment packages us usually high in sodium. Instead, you can make your own sauces, spice mixtures, or salad dressings.
- *Be mindful of the salty snacks*. These are the top contributors of excessive sodium levels in the body, like chips, pretzels, salted nuts, etc. You can look for low sodium alternatives and choose healthier snack options.

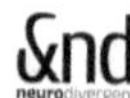

- *Hydration is a necessary measure.* Ven if you have had excess sodium intake, try drinking water throughout the day. This will no doubt make you urinate more, but that's only because you want that to happen. The more urine products, the more sodium excreted out.

It's high time you break free from this salty obsession of yours and give other flavors a chance. Combine salty flavor with other flavors and experience the culinary artistry. Trust me, there's a whole world of herbs, spices, seasoning and condiments waiting for you to give them a try.

Your Food Compass

Individualizing your diet means customizing a meal plan and some recipes according to your own needs so that you may get the nutrition that you require. Doesn't it sound great? You not only get to avoid the excess amount of food groups that your body doesn't require, but also stay healthy and nutritious. For that purpose, here are some strategies to help you with that:

- *Consider your goals* and needs, like weight management, handling any health condition, or simply athletic purposes. Such goals will be your nutritional compass and guide your towards an individualized diet.
- *Seek professional guidance* because you need the help of a pro to tell you what to eat and what not to eat. These medical professionals can help you get a customized diet plan tailored to your individual preferences and needs. Go to a nutritionist or a dietitian and get personalized recommendations based on your health status, lifestyle, and goals.
- *Listen to your body.* Pay attention to how a particular food makes you feel. Do you get a stomachache when you drink milk? Does your stomach hurt after eating bread? What happens when you eat sugars? What happens

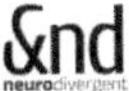

when you take spicy food? Notice any changes in energy levels, digestion, or overall well-being after consuming certain foods. This self-awareness can help you identify which foods work best for you.

- *Keeping a food journal* can allow you to keep track f the recipes, ingredients and products that you have added and incorporated, or avoided. This can provide valuable insights into your individual responses to different foods. You can start by trying new foods and recipes to expand your palate and find what you enjoy.
- *Prioritize nutrient-dense foods* by focusing on consuming a variety of nutrient-dense foods that provide essential vitamins, minerals, and antioxidants. Do not forget to include a balance of fruits, vegetables, whole grains, lean proteins, and healthy fats in your diet.
- *Consider food sensitivities and allergies* because of you suspect that you may have sensitivity to gluten, you have got to keep an eye out for gluten free foods. Maybe consider getting tested for sensitivities and allergies as well so that you may eliminate or reduce these foods from your diet to support your individual needs.
- *Adapt to your cultural preferences*. Respect and honor your heritage and personal values by including traditional or plant-based options that align with your beliefs. This way you develop a healthier relationship with food and make more conscious choices, end before you know it, you're practicing mindful eating.
- *Stay flexible* and keep in mind that your body preferences will change over time. It will not remain the same. For instance, you loved to eat spicy induna food during your college years – if you even went to college – but now that you're in your thirties, spicy food no longer agrees with you. So stay open to adjustments and modifications.

You must be thinking, why is Muneeba bothered so much, well you want to know what really irks me? The lack of mindfulness

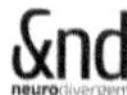

when it comes to eating. People should always take time to savor each and every bite, but instead, people like you are always scrolling though your phones, shoveling down food and rushing from one task to another. Appreciating the nourishment food provides is mindfulness.

It's just so frustrating. All the evidence is right in front of your eyes, staring in your face, and yet you choose to ignore it. I'm telling you; no one will suffer except for you. Unless you wake up, pay attention, and start making choices that'll support your overall well-being. Trust me it is not that complicated.

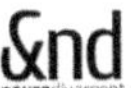

CHAPTER
5

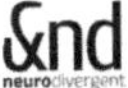

Part 1

To Meat or Not to Meat – The Great Diet Dilemma

Alright, brace yourselves for a riveting discussion. Have you ever heard about the animal-based diet and the plant-based diet? Well these are exactly what they sound like. The animal-based diet is all about animal-based foods like meat, poultry, fish, and seafood. These delightful creatures are the main source of protein and essential nutrients for all you meat enthusiasts out there. Oh, and did I mention carnivores have these amazing digestive systems specifically designed to process and extract nutrients from animal tissues? Yeah, that is how your body is made. Thus, the animal-based diet is also known as the carnivorous diet.

On the other hand, the plant-based diet includes foods like fruits, vegetables, grains, legumes, and nuts. Hold your applause, please. Herbivores, those plant-loving creatures, rely on these plant sources for protein, carbohydrates, vitamins, minerals, and even fiber. Oh, and they also have their own special digestive systems, all geared up to break down plant matter and extract nutrients with unparalleled efficiency. Which is why this plant based diet is also known as the herbivorous diet. Fascinating stuff, really.

Here's what I don't get; people go all the way towards either one of these extremes. Some might say that a carnivorous diet is the best food plan there is, while others may say that the

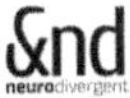

plant diet is the ideal way. We have to get through this dilemma together, so let's just end this food feud once and for all.

Predator's Digest

The carnivore diet is the latest fascination that has captured the attention of many people. Followers of this dietary approach passionately claim its multitude of health benefits and its unmatched nutritional completeness compared to other diets. It's crazy how strongly they believe in this. But of course, as with anything, there are those who criticize and highlight the potential for nutritional deficiencies and health complications. Let's delve into the most common concerns and misconceptions surrounding the carnivore diet. Time to dive into the depths of this divisive dietary trend and see if it truly lives up to its grand claims or if it's just another passing dietary craze.

Nutritional Stereotype: The fact that this diet doesn't include fruits or vegetables, or anything other than an animal-based food is one of the most common concerns about the carnivore diet. However, the supporters argue that the animal based food products like grass-fed meats, wild-caught fish etc., are nutrient dense and the also provide a wide variety of essential vitamins and minerals in their most natural and bioavailable forms.

It is important to know that the quality, quantity and the appropriate ratio of minerals and vitamins is more important than the type of food consumed. So to ensure that the nutrition intake is adequate, it's essential to have a plate full of a diverse range of animal based foods.

Toxicity Tales: Some critics claim that a diet consisting solely of animal based food products might lead to iron and vitamin A toxicity. All of the micronutrients that we consume work together in homeostasis, pulling and pushing each

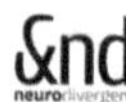

other to maintain a balance, so to avoid vitamin A toxicity, Vitamins K, E and D3 are consumed.

Although it is understandable that animal based diet is rich in iron, the human body is capable of regulating iron absorption using a hormone named as hepcidin. Basically, our liver helps in moving the iron, so it doesn't accumulate at toxic levels. There are many such natural mechanisms present to maintain the balance among the nutrient levels. Let me clear it up: if there are toxic levels of iron in the body, it doesn't mean that they're due to the high consumption of iron. It simply means that iron regulation has been compromised, and usually an underlying inflammation is the cause, and that is because the pathogenic bacteria responsible for the inflammation need iron to flourish too.

Cancer Concerns: It is also argued that risks of cancer are increased due to the consumption of only animal-based products like red meats. There are some studies that have been conducted which suggest a link between the intake of red meat, and an increased risk of certain cancers, but it is necessary to realize that a study might not have a statistically accurate results. Also, the quality of the meat consumed is the important factor here. Grass-fed, and Pasteur-raised meats have lesser harmful chemical compounds than their conventionally raised counterparts, and the former are more nutrient dense than the latter as well. If you don't understand or believe all this, shake your common sense and ask yourself: Did the food that made us evolve over millions of years suddenly cause cancer?

Fiber Fallacy: A key point of this contention lies in the functions of dietary fibers, serving as one of the strongest opposing arguments. I mean, everyone knows that fibers are important for maintaining a healthy digestive tract. But the proponents of the carnivore diet state that fibers

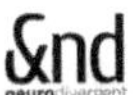

are not a requirement for a healthy diet. Instead, followers of this duet approach actually find their digestive system improving as soon as they leave the plant based diets, claiming that the vegetarian foods cause bloating, gas, etc. Moreover, the advocates of the carnivorous diet claim that consuming adequate amount of water is good enough for the bowel functioning. The only reasons you might have digestive issues on a carnivore diet are perhaps at the beginning. This is because your body is getting used to foods you haven't eaten before or haven't eaten in such quantities.

Fact-Checked and Research-Backed: Let's break it down with science, because you somehow consider my research-backed knowledge as empty statements and have always demanded a scientific justification. And don't worry, I'm not going to take this assumption personal, so here's something for you to digest:

If we take a look at the ancestral context of the animal-based diet, it will prove that our ancestors did not have access to vegetables and fruits of all the seasons over the years. That deprivation lead to the consumption of nutrient dense animal foods to achieve a complete and balanced consumption of vitamins and minerals. Other than that, common concern regarding the carnivore diet is the deficiency of vitamin C in meat products. Although fruits and vegetables are rich in vitamin C, meat also contains this vitamin, albeit in lesser concentration than the fruits. Moreover, some of the organs are nutritionally complete, which means that they provide vitamins – both water soluble and fat soluble – as well as the essential minerals. Let me give you an example: the liver contains surplus amounts of Vitamin E and copper, while caviar, made from the roe of fish, contains exceptionally high concentrations of omega-3 fatty acids.

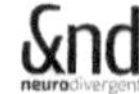

Thoughts and Flavors Combined: When I first started the carnivore diet, I went through diarrhea, which went on for two days. It's like leaving a car in the garage without using it for years. Of course, it will most definitely be difficult to start. But I knew that my body would get used to this in a few days. The thing is, people like you have one meal, feel strange, and conclude that this is not for you. To sum it all up, it is safe to say that the carnivorous diet is fully capable of providing a balanced combination of nutrients , even though a wide variety of food is not on the plate. The main thing to focus on is the consumption of only the nutrient-rich animal-based foods which contains the necessary minerals and vitamins for the body's optimal growth and overall health.

Choosing to embark on a carnivore diet, much like any dietary pathway, should be a conscious decision driven by personal preferences, health requirements, and professional medical advice. It seems so straightforward, doesn't it? This wisdom rings true for any dietary or lifestyle choices we make. So, if you're aligning yourself with the carnivore lifestyle, be prepared to dance with steaks, waltz with chicken breasts, and tango with a fish or two. But in this gastronomic ballroom, it's not just about the partners you choose, but how well-groomed they are. Grass-fed, pasture-raised, wild-caught - we're talking about the créme de la créme of the meat world for our carnivorous soiree.

However, let's open the curtain a bit on our meaty performers. Whether you're a plant lover or a meat aficionado, the harsh truth is that the real puppet master behind our food choices is the colossal industry, often manipulating the strings with hormones, herbicides, and other additives. Sometimes the labels and buzzwords like "eco" and "organic" are more marketing strategies than they are guarantees of better food. They parade around in fancy suits - grass-fed this, pasture-raised that - but under the surface, the story isn't always as it

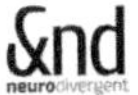

seems. While we're here primarily to talk about nutrition and diet, it's worth noting that the industry's machinations could fill another book entirely. Consider this a little spoiler from your friendly neighborhood author - we might not be able to control the entire show, but we can certainly choose which puppet we want to dance with.

"But,–" Stop.

I am on my way to the plant-based diet even before you started to whine. Have some patience my friend and let's talk about the other side of the picture.

Harvesting Health

In contrast to the animal-diet, the plant-diet is a dietary approach that is all about consuming plant-based food products and minimizing – eventually, eliminating – all animal-based food products. It basically revolves around the idea of embracing whole grains, fruits, vegetables, legumes, nuts, and seeds as the foundation of one's meals.

Just like the followers of the carnivore diet, the advocates of the herbivore diet emphasize on the potential benefits this approach offers, such as the increased intake of dietary fiber, vitamins, minerals, and antioxidants may help lower the risk of chronic diseases, including heart disease, diabetes, and certain cancers. Moreover, proponents assert that by reducing reliance on animal products, the plant-based diet can have positive impacts on the environment and animal welfare. To sum it all up, the vegan lifestyle promotes the consumption of nutrient-rich plant foods, highlighting their benefits for overall health and well-being.

But let's be real here for a minute. Can a diet consisting solely of plants really provide everything our bodies need? Are we

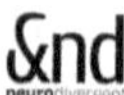

supposed to ignore the cravings for a juicy steak or succulent chicken, just to munch on a kale leaf? Are you really doomed if you dare to stray from their green gospel?

"Plants are not as innocent as they seem"

In a thought-provoking lecture by Dr. Anthony Chaffee, a neurosurgeon and advocate of the carnivore diet, stated that plants produce various toxins and carcinogenic compounds. This controversial statement sparked a heated debate within the nutrition community, challenging the belief that plant-based diets are the healthiest option for humans. Have you ever heard about *antinutrients*?

Antinutrients are naturally occurring compounds found in certain plant-based foods that can interfere with the absorption or utilization of nutrients in the body. These antinutrients act as a defense mechanism against predators. Antinutrients can bind to minerals, impair digestive enzymes, or interfere with the absorption of certain vitamins. Some examples of antinutrients found in plant-based foods include:

- **Glucosinolates:** Present in broccoli, cabbage, kale etc. These antinutrients are also known as *goitrogens* can interfere and prevent the absorption of iodine. This eventually leads to goiter.

- **Lectins, and Saponins:** Present in legumes (like beans, peanuts) and whole grains.
  These can interfere with the absorption of various minerals like iron, zinc, phosphorous, calcium.

- **Oxalates:** Present in green leafy vegetables, nuts etc.
  Oxalates inhibit the absorption of calcium by binding to it.

- **Tannins:** Present in tea and coffee.
  Tannins are known for causing a decrease in the iron absorption.

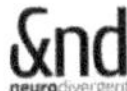

Don't panic yet. It's worth noting that not all antinutrients have negative effects on health. In fact, some may have potential health benefits, such as antioxidant and anticancer properties. Additionally, many antinutrients can be reduced or eliminated through proper food preparation methods like soaking, fermenting, cooking, or sprouting.

But, while many experts argue that these antinutrients are present in such small amounts that they do not pose a significant health risk, Dr. Chaffee believes that their cumulative effects can be harmful, particularly for those who rely heavily on plant-based diets. It's a neither-nor kind of a situation.

"The Vegetarian Myth"

"The Vegetarian Myth" is a book written by a former vegetarian and vegan of 20 years, Lierre Keith, and it also explores the potential dangers of plant-based diets. Keith exposes the health risks she experienced and the fallacies she encountered during her journey through veganism and vegetarianism. Let me share parts of her agonizing journey with you.

Just six weeks into her veganism, she got hypoglycemia. And she didn't realize what it was called for 18 years. By then, hypoglycemia had become a part of her life. Three months into her vegan diet, Keith stopped menstruating. She admits that she should have known by then that something was off. Not only was she exhausted all the time, but she also suffered from an ever-present cold. Which also had an adverse effect on her skin. At the age of twenty-four, she suffered from gastroparesis. Keith was not properly diagnosed or treated until she was thirty-eight. And it was a doctor that specifically worked with recovering vegans. Her story only gets worse from here. Two years into her vegan hood, her health failed catastrophically. Keith developed a

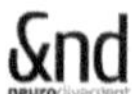

degenerative joint disease which started out as a dull pain and after a few months ended up feeling like a shrapnel in her spine. She describes her Degenerative Disc Disease as a spine that "looks like a sky-diving accident". The episodes of anxiety, and the family history of depression didn't do her any good either. And malnutrition was the last thing that she needed.

After changing her diet and incorporating grass-fed animal based food products into her meals, she felt like some damage has been compensated. Her insulin levels are getting back to normal; pain levels have been slightly decreased, she doesn't miss a period, and as far as she takes her daily medication, her stomach is okay as well. Not only this, but she has also gotten some control over her depression. She feels happier and gratuitous.

"Some days breathing takes more energy than I have." Says Keith. "You're allowed to learn from my mistakes."

It seems like everyone is jumping on the plant-based bandwagon these days, singing praises about how amazing it is for your health and the environment. Sure, there may be some benefits associated with a plant-based diet, like a reduced risk of chronic diseases and improved heart health. But seriously, we need to stop pretending that it's the only way to go. So, go ahead and embrace your plant-based lifestyle if that's what you're into.

But, like any dietary approach, it is crucial for you to consider various perspectives and find a balance that works best for you. While Dr. Chaffee's lecture and Keith's book present thought-provoking arguments against plant-based diets, it is essential to remember that there are countless studies and health professionals who advocate for the benefits of a balanced plant-based diet. It is also important to consult with

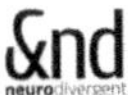

a healthcare professional, such as a nutritionist or a dietitian, before making significant changes to one's diet.

There are plenty of other dietary choices that can also provide health benefits. And let's not forget that not all plant-based diets are created equal. It's important to ensure that a plant-based diet is well-planned, balanced, and meets all your nutrient needs so let's not act like it's the holy grail of nutrition. There are other options out there, and it's important to consider them too.

As the Dust Settles, We Tie Up the Loose Ends

Both of these diets, as you can see, are compatible with human beings as we are provided with both kinds of facilities. It's like arguing over whether we're meant to eat apples or oranges. Well, newsflash: we're adaptable beings, capable of deriving nutrition from a wide range of food sources.

Our bodies have evolved to handle both plant-based and animal-based foods. There are some people who insist that our teeth and digestive systems prove we're herbivores. Oh, really? Have they ever seen our canine teeth? Yes, we have them, and they're designed for tearing and ripping flesh. We have stomach acid strong enough to break down animal proteins, and our intestines are versatile enough to handle both plant fibers and animal fats. It's almost as if we're adaptable omnivores or something. You just need to make sure you get enough nutrients and manage your oh-so-specific health concerns. Because even though one diet may not be the right choice for everyone - surprise, surprise - some people may actually find it beneficial and align it perfectly with their nutritional needs and goals. The Japanese diet is worth mentioning here.

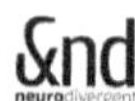

The Power of *Washoku*

The Japanese are infamous for their knack for living long and living well. Seriously, they've got it going on. With their sky-high life expectancies, they've practically cracked the code to eternal youth. And guess what? It's all about their diet. A key aspect of their dietary habits is the emphasis on fresh, seasonal, and locally sourced products. Studies have shown that the traditional Japanese diet, rich in fish, vegetables, and fermented foods, contributes to their overall health and longevity.

The National Center for Global Health and Medicine conducted a study in Tokyo which concluded that those participants who were sticking to the Japanese diet, had a much lower risk of cardiovascular diseases and overall mortality. The focus on fresh, nutrient-dense, and minimally processed foods in the Japanese diet is believed to be a significant factor in their extended lifespans.

Furthermore, the principle for the Japanese diet is to listen to their bodies. The human body is incredibly intelligent and has an innate ability to signal what it needs in terms of nutrients and nourishment. This is evidence that no matter what the diet approach is, as long as you consume fresh, minimally unprocessed and nutrient-dense foods, and ensure that you are providing your body with the essential nutrients, you'll achieve optimum health and vitality.

If we dig deep and think about why some groups do not prefer meat or animal based diets, we come to the conclusion that they desire a healthier lifestyle. But if we really think about *why* a healthier lifestyle is desired, the answer is simple: people don't want to go early. Longevity of life is the ultimate goal here and this reminds me of a book I read, The Blue Zones.

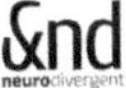

Part 2

The Blue Zones:
The (Misleading) Diet
of Longevity

We have often been sold the idea of 'Blue Zones' by various media outlets – the five regions of the world with the highest concentration of centenarians per inhabitant. These regions are held as the model to emulate for a long and quality life. The five regions in question are Sardinia (Italy), Okinawa (Japan), Nicoya (Costa Rica), Icaria (Greece), and Loma Linda (California).

The author who popularized this idea has written ten books on the subject, yet he has neglected to mention key information that we'll explore today. If he had included these insights, perhaps the force with which the media promotes the diet based on these areas of the world might have been significantly weakened.

What do Blue Zone Centenarians Really Eat?

A key question that arises is, "What do the centenarians of the Blue Zones actually eat?" The answer to this query can be gleaned by observing the types of diets and foods that are promoted by the media and governments.

Take for example Bryan Johnson, a multimillionaire who reportedly spends two million dollars a year in an attempt

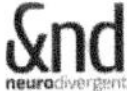

to reverse his biological age. Despite his desire for longevity, Johnson's lifestyle – consisting of swallowing dozens of pills each morning, being enslaved by his habits, and consuming over 30kg of vegetables monthly – appears quite undesirable, irrespective of the possibility of living up to 150 years.

Johnson is not the only one to have swallowed the narrative that consuming vegetables will extend our lifespan. Interestingly, even centenarians from the Blue Zones don't necessarily live longer due to consuming more vegetables.

The Dirty Secret of Blue Zones

The inconvenient truth about the Blue Zones is that their populations are neither vegan nor vegetarian, contrary to popular belief. One may wonder why it is often reported that they consume many plants and why only five Blue Zones are spoken about when there are other populations in the world that also have a considerable number of centenarians. Why were societies with even more centenarians than the official Blue Zones not included?

Why don't we talk about Hong Kong, where each person consumes an average of 664 grams of meat a day, making it the second country in the world with the highest life expectancy? Moreover, it is a country that spends relatively little on healthcare yet ranks high as one of the most intelligent societies in the world. Let's dive in.

Origin of the Blue Zones

The term "Blue Zones" was popularized by Dan Buettner, a best-selling author of the New York Times. The idea of living 100 years or more is certainly appealing, hence longevity is a concept that sells well. Buettner found great success with

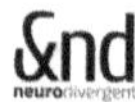

this narrative, publishing over ten books, all revolving around the Blue Zones. His businesses also focus primarily on this concept.

Interestingly, in one interview, Buettner candidly shared that he had invested in companies that produce lab-grown meat, which coincidentally aligns with the parts of the Blue Zones' diet he promotes.

The Problem with the Blue Zones

Buettner's narrative is eerily reminiscent of Ancel Keys, who decided not to include many other countries in his list, leaving only a list of seven countries that fit his narrative that cholesterol was bad.

Keys designed his study with a clear bias, cherry-picking certain areas of the world that fit his belief that cholesterol was bad. This is an example of epidemiology, which is fundamentally observational and not clinical. In this context, many factors such as lifestyle, exercise, healthcare quality, food quality, and social relationships are often ignored.

The True Diet of the Five Blue Zones

The diet of individuals residing in the Blue Zones has been speculated to be 95% to 100% plant-based (vegan). However, this is not the truth. Even Buettner, the proponent of this misguided idea, admitted in an interview that they do consume meat.

To fully understand, we need to look at each of the five populations individually, along with an extra longevity hotspot closer to home, which surprisingly didn't make the list.

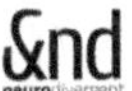

Sardinia, Italy

People from Sardinia, one of the official Blue Zones, consume more meat than the average Western diet, though the percentage difference isn't dramatic.

So, why are they healthier than the rest of the world? The answer lies in the quality of their food. Blue Zone populations do not live in large cities. They are rural folk, who typically do not purchase cheap, factory-farmed meat or consume homogenized, pasteurized milk. Instead, they consume quality produce. They drink wholesome milk and eat animals that have freely roamed their land.

This doesn't mean they only consume animal products. They also consume vegetables and grains, but these are prepared and cooked traditionally and are of much higher quality than industrially produced versions.

These traditional meals are not only nutritionally dense but are also much less inflammatory than the average diet in the developed world. As such, it is crucial to bear in mind that I am talking about the traditional diets of the Blue Zones. Modern society may well be influencing the consumption habits of the newer generations in these areas.

But this gives us a glimpse into the real secret of the Blue Zones: It's not about cutting out entire food groups or living on a diet of raw vegetables. Instead, it's about eating quality, traditionally prepared food, maintaining strong social bonds, and living an active, meaningful life. These are the true keys to longevity that we should be taking from the Blue Zones.

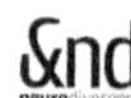

Okinawa, Japan

Something similar happens with the people of Okinawa. "But wait, Muneeba, didn't they get most of their calories from sweet potatoes?"

Well, not exactly.

In a paper analyzing 94 centenarian men in Japan, a higher proportion of animal food was seen than the average Japanese person. "The increase in the intake of milk, fats, and oils have healthy effects on their longevity," said the paper. In fact, I quote verbatim:

"Unexpectedly, we found no vegetarians among the centenarians."

What people don't know is that the true Okinawan diet is centered around meat. Especially pork, but all you hear about is their consumption of sweet potatoes.

While nearly 70% of the population in Japan is Buddhist, it is not the case in Okinawa, which allows them to eat meat. And they certainly do eat meat.

The Okinawa Blue Zone study was carried out in 1949, and while traditionally this area cared for a huge population of pigs on its island, the number of pigs was very low at the time of the study because World War II had just ended. It was not until 1960 that the pig population in Okinawa regained the number it had lost during the war.

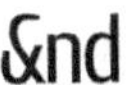

Nicoya, Costa Rica

What's going on in Nicoya, Costa Rica? The average man in Nicoya is 7 times more likely to be a centenarian than the average Japanese man. As we have just seen, Japan is one of the societies with the longest life expectancy. People in Nicoya consume large amounts of fish, poultry, eggs, even turtles and many types of animals in their hunts, according to various reports.

A 109-year-old lady described her favorite dish as pork leg, cooked with liver, kidney, ear, brain, and heart.

The carnivorous diet of only meat was popular long before the internet was invented, and although they surely include some vegetables, they are not full of pesticides and they do not make up the majority of their calories as is happening with current Western diets, or with the false longevity diet sold in these books.

It is known that this area of Costa Rica cooks with more animal fat than vegetable compared to the rest of the Costa Rican population.

Ikaria, Greece

In the case of the Ikarians, with 1 in 3 reaching 90 years of age, despite not consuming much grass-fed meat, they do consume fish.

They usually have a late breakfast (intermittent fasting?) consisting of pasture-fed goat yogurt or cheese, some vegetables with generous amounts of olive oil.

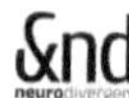

Locally caught fish is consumed practically every day, and a goat or pig is sacrificed once a week (which provided meat for several days depending on the family).

Loma Linda, California

Four of the five sites have similar percentages of animal product consumption to Spain in general or to the world.

But what about Loma Linda, California, where the religious people of the **Seventh Day Adventist** Church do not eat meat? These people are the only vegetarians on the official list of blue zones, but is it the diet or the fact of not eating meat that makes them live so long?

Loma Linda, California is the only Blue Zone in the United States and has a notably high concentration of Seventh-day Adventists. This religious group practices a variety of healthy habits that contribute to their long lives. They don't drink or smoke, they do a lot of exercises, have a purpose, a very strong social circle.

The Adventist Health Studies, a long-term series of studies exploring the health and lifestyle habits of Seventh-day Adventists in the U.S and Canada, have found that vegetarian Adventists tend to live longer than their non-vegetarian counterparts. These studies, however, also take into account other aspects of the Adventist lifestyle that contribute to their longevity.

Beyond diet, the Seventh-day Adventist lifestyle includes regular physical activity, abstaining from smoking and alcohol, maintaining a healthy body weight, and strong community connections. They also emphasize the importance of rest, particularly observing a 24-hour Sabbath each week, which can contribute to reduced stress and improved mental health.

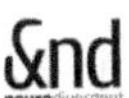

These different elements of the Adventist lifestyle might contribute collectively to their longer lifespans. So while the vegetarian diet followed by many in Loma Linda is certainly a significant aspect, it's not the only factor at play. It's crucial to consider the holistic approach that the Adventist community takes towards health and wellness.

In conclusion, the Blue Zones offer compelling examples of lifestyle and dietary practices that contribute to longer, healthier lives. It's important to remember that these practices aren't strictly about diet. Regular physical activity, strong social connections, a sense of purpose and belonging, and other lifestyle factors are just as crucial to longevity. It's the combination of all these factors that seems to be the true secret to the longevity seen in these regions.

You may have noticed that alongside a good diet, the routine of these centenarians is worth mentioning. Mainly all the people in those Blue Zones have an active lifestyle and we all know that regular exercise is essential for sound body and sound mind. So let's have a look at that.

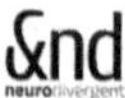

CHAPTER
6

Part 1

FIT - Fueling Incredible Transformations

Picture yourself standing at the foot of a towering mountain. Its peak vanishes into the clouds, and the path winding up its side appears steep, rugged, and long. This mountain symbolizes your fitness journey. Yes, it might seem daunting at first, but remember that every long journey begins with a single step. While 80% of the battle lies in your diet, let's gear up to conquer the remaining 20% – exercise.

As Dr David Perlmutter MD would say, physical activity, particularly aerobic exercise, is not just beneficial for the body; it has profound effects on the brain too. It plays a significant role in epigenetics, which is the study of changes in gene expression. Exercise activates genes associated with longevity and the gene responsible for the production of a protein called Brain-Derived Neurotrophic Factor (BDNF), which is often referred to as the brain's growth hormone. Studies have demonstrated that aerobic exercise can reverse memory decline in elderly individuals and stimulate the growth of new brain cells in the hippocampus, a brain region crucial for memory and learning.

It's been proposed that our prehistoric ancestors' ability to outpace predators and catch prey led to the survival of the fittest. This suggests that we may have inherited genes favoring endurance and athleticism. This theory underscores

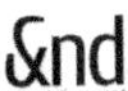

the importance of staying active in preserving our health and cognitive abilities.

To be honest, I had no clue which exercises suit me, what time was the most optimum time for exercise, and what should be the duration of my routine, but I do know this: never commit to something long term without any scientific backup, or researched logic. Here, we're going to decode some core principles of fitness, seasoned with a generous dose of scientific evidence and practical tips. Ready to break a sweat? Let's go!

Pushing Towards Muscular Failure

"Intensity with Sensibility"

As you lift, there comes a point where your muscles scream in protest, a moment when you feel you couldn't possibly do another rep. That's muscular failure. But should you regularly train to this extreme? Research suggests that's not necessary. A study published in the Journal of Strength and Conditioning Research found that participants who trained to failure across three sets had no significant increase in muscle size compared to those who stopped short of failure. The takeaway? Push your limits, but don't consistently hit muscular failure. Listen to your body; when your reps significantly slow down, it's time to hit pause.

Overtraining and Fatigue

"Pace your Race"

Did you know that while you work out, you're breaking your muscle fibers down? It's during the rest period that your body repairs these fibers, making them stronger. However, if you consistently push your body to its limits without allowing

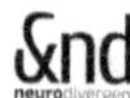

sufficient recovery time, it's like trying to build a skyscraper on shaky foundations. In 2002, a study published in the Journal of Applied Physiology showed that overtraining could lead to a decrease in performance and muscle mass. The solution? Respect your body's recovery process. After a heavy workout, ensure you get adequate sleep and nutrition to aid recovery.

Training Frequency and Rest Periods

"The Art of Timing"

How often should you train a muscle group? A study in the Journal of Strength and Conditioning Research suggests training each muscle group twice a week for optimal muscle growth. But remember, your body isn't a machine. It needs time to recover between sets. The American College of Sports Medicine recommends a rest period of 2-3 minutes between each set for optimal strength gains. And if your goal is hypertrophy, you might need to tweak this depending on your routine and how your body feels.

Hypertrophy Through Stretching and Mind-Muscle Connection

"Stretch, Feel, Grow"

When you perform an exercise, focusing on the muscle you're working. The mind-muscle connection can amplify your results. A study in the European Journal of Sports Science showed that participants who focused on their muscles during workouts experienced greater muscle activity. Additionally, stretching a muscle under tension can stimulate muscle growth. For example, when doing bicep curls, let your arm fully extend at the bottom to get a good stretch, and focus on your bicep as you curl the weight.

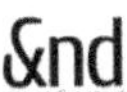

Addressing Stress, Cortisol, and Exercise

"Finding Calm in the Storm"

Exercise raises cortisol, the body's "stress hormone," but don't let that deter you. A temporary spike in cortisol from a rigorous workout won't disintegrate your hard-earned muscles. In fact, a study published in the Journal of Endocrinology indicates that this cortisol surge might be beneficial by improving energy utilization and increasing stress resistance.

However, persistent high levels of cortisol, due to chronic stress or overtraining, can be a roadblock to muscle gain. In an enlightening study in the Journal of Strength and Conditioning Research, excessive cortisol was associated with reduced muscle strength and mass. So, take it easy, champ! Make sure your training regimen allows ample time for recovery and relaxation. A balanced lifestyle, complete with healthy nutrition, sound sleep, and mindful relaxation, can help keep cortisol levels under control.

Building Habits for Long-Term Success

"Consistency is Key"

Transforming your physique is akin to sculpting a masterpiece – it takes time, patience, and consistent effort. While we can always draw inspiration from the bodies of athletes and bodybuilders, remember that these impressive physiques are built upon years of consistent training and disciplined lifestyle. The journey towards your fitness goal is more like a marathon rather than a sprint.

One method to foster consistency in your exercise routine is to incorporate exercises you enjoy. A meta-analysis published in the Journal of Behavioral Medicine suggests that intrinsic

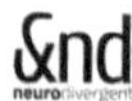

motivation – doing something because you find it enjoyable or rewarding – is a powerful driver of long-term adherence to exercise.

Savor the Journey

Building muscle is a marathon, not a sprint. As with any long journey, there will be tough climbs, easy plains, thrilling highs, and challenging lows. It's important to keep going, step by step, with determination and discipline. At times, you may feel impatient, but remember that the path to your dream physique is not straight but a winding road filled with valuable lessons. Listen to your body, respect its limits, and fuel it with nutritious food. With the right approach and a resilient spirit, you can conquer that towering mountain. As the saying goes, "Rome wasn't built in a day," and neither will your dream physique be.

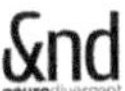

Part 2

The Fitness Formula: Unlocking Your Personalized Workout Routine

I cannot emphasize the importance of *regular* exercise enough. Your weight and your physique should not just be about you trying to fit into your favorite pair of jeans, or getting ready for Summer where you have a beach-ready body. In fact, exercise should be about your lifestyle, how important is exercise to unlock a healthier and more fulfilling life. I realize how necessary it is to delve into the transformative benefits of *regular* exercise in this book, after all it is a matter of your physical and mental well-being.

I personally (and very strongly) believe in the 'regular' part of regular exercise. And that is because there is no use of exercising once in a blue moon. Imagine you exercise only once a month. What good would it do to your body? What changes do you think it'll bring? Obviously apart from the muscle cramps, nothing. When you want to achieve a healthy lifestyle, and want to maintain your fitness, you must teach yourself patience and consistency. Mark my words: *regular* exercise is an indisputable and non-negotiable price for a healthy existence. It's not some optional add-on; it's an absolute must.

Let's suppose that you have started going to the gym for consistent and regular exercise. I can understand it might be a bit hard to imagine, but give it a try, I believe in you.

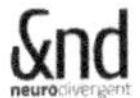

I'll wait a little longer.

Okay, now that I have successfully changed your imaginary routine, and you have started going to the gym every week, there are some of the changes that your body will go through. Internally, your cardiovascular system will be fortified, which means that your heart will be pumping with power. Your muscular system, especially the skeletal muscles will be stronger, more toned, and then there will be no stopping you. You'll not only achieve flexibility and endurance, but also achieve a sound mind. Regular exercise will become your fortress against stress, anxiety, and depression, unveiling a sharper mind and heightened cognitive abilities. And just like a cherry on top, regular exercise will protect you from chronic diseases like heart conditions, diabetes, cancers even. You've got to admit that exercise is the very bedrock of a vibrant and spirited life.

Do you remember how Sarah started to go to the gym as well? Well, things weren't too easy for her when the gyms were shut down due to the COVID-19 lockdown. Sarah lost her routine, and she began to face some losses. According to an associate professor Rob Robergs, who is an exercise physiologist in the Queensland University of Technology, the losses are ten times faster than the gains as the body is constantly trying to conserve energy. And Sarah knew that. She was aware that she is losing all her benefits from her training.

"Have I lost my muscle?" She began over thinking. "How long till I am out of shape?"

Within the first few days, she noticed that her heart rate increased. This usually happens because of the fact that the heart loses its endurance. After the first few weeks, her body went through biological changes like changes in her muscle size, and that eventually led towards weight gain. After a

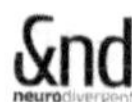

few months, which is considered as a long-term break from exercise and training, Sarah felt alarmed when she was out of breath during her trip to the grocery store. She used to be out of breath before her exercise routine started, but being in the same situation at that moment, realization dawned upon her that she is back to square one.

Somehow she found a way to exercise at home. I mean, all she did while working from home was eat, sit in front of her laptop, make something to eat, and then eat it, maybe clean the house, and eventually go to bed, where she slept only after surfing through the internet for a few hours. All the while, watching YouTube videos and tutorials on exercises at home. Because apparently at-home workouts were famous all of a sudden. Sarah realized one definite thing, which initially was the reason of her motivation for at-home workouts:

"I don't need gym equipment for my workouts."

Yoga, strength training and cardio are some of the types of exercises that you can easily do at home, on your own, in your own time. And that's what Sarah chose. She knew that she needed to incorporate all these three categories of exercises in order to achieve ultimate fitness. I mean, if you think about it, it's a smart plan. You might be able to master a handstand, but at the same time you might also run out of break after running a kilometer or so. She knew that total body fitness is always achieved by a combination of exercises that improve your strength, endurance, flexibility, power, and balance. She initially focused on beginner exercises and developing a routine, deciding that a 10-15 minute workout would be enough, as she had read in a study from the Journal of American Heart Association that short bursts of 10-minute exercise is just as fruitful for one's health as the longer workouts. The key is to plan proper sessions and space them throughout the week, giving yourself enough time to rest. There are certain websites

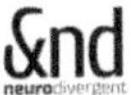

that helped Sarah figure out the exercises she needs to do and with all that in mind, she created a sample plan for her training. Here's what it looked like:

Monday:

- 20 minutes of weight training- focusing on her upper body
- 20 minutes on the treadmill for a steady state cardio (it is important to realize that a treadmill is not a necessary. Sarah had the limitation of a COVID lockdown, otherwise sh would have gone for a run)
- 20 minutes for yoga

Tuesday:

- 20 minutes of weight training- focusing on her lower body
- 20 minutes of sets of High Intensity Interval Training, or HIIT cardio, which includes short and intense exercises like jumping jacks, pushups, lunges, sprints, squats etc.
- 20 minutes for yoga

Wednesday:

- 1 hour of yoga poses

Thursday:

- Same as her Monday routine

Friday:

- Same as her Tuesday routine

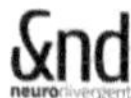

Saturday:

- Going for a walk, cleaning the house, grocery shopping, basically an activity that kept Sarah up and going on her feet.

Sunday:

- Rest, as resting is extremely important for long term routines.

If you plan on following Sarah's routine, I must advice you to stop, think, research, and then start working out. Because it is crucial that you go with what's best for you. Your body's goals may not be the same as those of Sarah's. Besides, if you're a newbie, you most definitely need a plan for beginners. Sarah's plan was just to maintain her routine, as she had been going to the gym to train. You can start by incorporating regular exercise in 2 or 3 days of the week first (with 2 days of cardio), then increase the frequency of your workouts to 3 to 4 days in a week (with 3 days of cardio), and then when you feel like leveling up, you may incorporate 5 – 6 weeks (with 3 days of cardio, and 1 day off, just like how Sarah did).

And this is why I am not going to give out a universal exercise plan or a general training workout routine for you. You've got to focus in individualizing a plan that is based on your body goals, whether you want to lose weight or gain muscle. I'm not saying that you hire a personal trainer (I'm also not saying it's a bad idea either, I mean, if you can afford a personal trainer then good for you, go for it) but for personalizing your own workout routine, notice what your body needs. Do you have lower belly fat? Are your arms your problematic areas? Do you think your legs are too skinny? Are you embarrassed from your de-shaped behind? Ask yourself these questions are you'll be one step closer to individualizing a training plan.

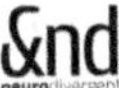

From Rust to Resilience

Once Sarah started to get back on track with her fitness plan, she started to feel some changes. On her first day back, she felt breathless, clumsy and exhausted. But she knew that the first workout was never going to satisfy her with a sense of accomplishment when she had discussed her situation with Iris. Robergs explains that your brain has to coordinate these new nerve patterns and that is why one may also feel mentally exhausted and fatigued. The next day, she felt her muscles ache which is explained by Robergs as DOMS or delayed onset muscle soreness that happens due to such contraction and relaxation of muscles that is enough to cause micro tears in the muscles. Stairs weren't her friends for days. Iris had informed her about DOMS, but she also warned her that if she was unable to sit without flinching with pain, she has overdone her exercise. The best way to get rid of the soreness is with movement. Sarah never stopped doing her house chores even with her muscles being sore. When she first started going to the gym, pre-COVID, she would often get a massage for her soreness but that was not an option anymore. At the end of her first week, Sarah felt the familiar sense of accomplishment. Those were her endorphins – the happy hormones. She wasn't sore anymore, and she realized that she was energetic and had a need to do more. Sam Rooney from Sydney's Ion Training, also an exercise physiologist, explains that the mitochondria – famously known as the powerhouse of the cell – multiples, hence the energy surge. After a month of her regular exercises, Sarah noticed improvements in her strength and fitness. She built up endurance and tolerance and noticed that her body doesn't take much time to recover from any kind of problematic situation. Be it physical or mental. Sarah observed that she had started sweating more as well. And that was a relief.

You might be wondering how is it a relief to sweat more.

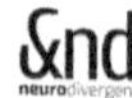

Sweat contains water and electrolytes – which is why we need to stay hydrated and make sure our electrolyte balance isn't fluctuating – but other than that it also contains some bacteria, which are the main reason why sweat isn't pleasant to the olfactory senses. But there is one other sweat component that acts an advocate to the fact that sweating is beneficial; that component is toxins. Liver and kidneys do the major detoxification of our bodies but sweating also helps in the process. The more toxins that are released from the body, the healthier we will be. Now if that clever little brain of yours tries to find out easy ways to sweat, keep in mind that it doesn't work like that. It's the activity that makes sweating healthy or harmful.

Home Sweet Gym

To make her workouts effective and her routine strict, Sarah kept a few things in mind. These are basically some tips that you should also keep in mind when you exercise, that is, *if* you ever decide to get up and be healthy:

- Choose a workout space that will allow you to easily practice your poses and exercises without bumping into furniture or breaking any vases.
- Get a good yoga mat as it protects your joints and bones, it protects the floor (like when you work with dumbbells, and you accidently drop one. No? Never happed to you? It's only me? Okay) and it also give you a good grip when you want to stay locked in, in a stable position.
- Always warm up. Walking is an excellent way to warm up. Warming up loosens up your muscles, increases your hart rate for maximum oxygen flow to the muscles, and primes the nerves for an improved movement efficiency. Just basically getting your body ready for the workout.
- Always cool down after every workout. Stretching is an excellent way to cool down. Cool down after exercise

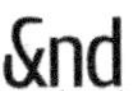

helps in recovering your heart rate and blood pressure gradually.
- Remember to breath. Never hold your breath during any exercise, as inhaling and exhaling flushes your muscles with oxygen.
- Always give your muscles some time off.

I want to add in a precaution for you; if you experience any pain or discomfort especially the ones that do not go away, you need to seek professional healthcare. If you sustain a head injury you should immediately go to a doctor, even if your head appears fine. Your safety should be your top priority. And it is with a disappointed sigh that I write this precaution for you because I knew that you had to be told about this. Moreover, always remember that exercise, diet, and proper rest, these go hand-in-hand, and this is something you need to learn how to balance.

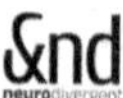

CHAPTER
7

Stressful Days, Restless Nights: Balancing Your Diet Amidst Life's Challenges

Ah yes. Sleep. The elusive elixir of life that seems to evade so many. I really want to emphasize on the impact sleep has on your health. It's quite funny when you think about how something so vital for our health and well-being can be so easily dismissed and taken for granted. Let me clarify this for you specifically; sleep is not just some luxury reserved for the weak or the lazy. No, my friend, it is an absolute necessity for our physical and mental health.

You need to have a conceptual understanding of the fact that sleep is when your body works its magic, it repairs and rejuvenates your body and makes sure that when you wake up, you feel like the best version of yourself. But I get the realty, in the fast pace of your routine and modern life, you barely find time to stop, rest and relax, and in return, getting a good night's sleep on a regular basis seems like a dream.

The Sleep Equation

If you do get a good eight hours of sleep and still do not feel refreshed, well, Dr. Marishka Brown, a sleep expert, will tell you that there's more to a good sleep than the hours you've spent in bed. The sleep equation includes three variables: the quantity of sleep, the quality of sleep and consistency of sleep. But here's the kicker: if you don't prioritize all these three variables of sleep, you're setting yourself up for a whole starter-pack of issues.

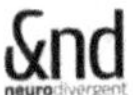

The Quantity Quotient

Look, I get it. Life is busy, and there are a million and one things demanding your attention. But let me tell you, sacrificing your sleep is a grave mistake. These are some serious physiological and psychological effects that sleep deprivation can cause like impairment of memory – long term and short term, both – poor judgement, decreased creativity (the last thing you needed), poor concentration and liable emotions. Moreover depression and anxiety are pretty common among individuals who have a sleep of less than 6 hours. Now, I am not here to lecture you on how you need to sleep for at least 6 to 8 hours a day, rather I am here to enlighten you on its impact on your health.

Researchers have managed to link psychological problems with sleep deprivation, like poor decision making skills, cognitive impairment, altered moods. Moreover, scientists have also gained evidence that ties physiological functions of the body to sleep quantity. For instance, if you suffer from lack of sleep, you may also have a detrimental effect on your immune system. Insufficient sleep is equal to a decrease in the production of antibodies and T-Lymphocytes (a type of immune cell) Not only will this increase the chances of an infection in the body, but you know how our body creates cancerous cells, and all the while our immune system gets rid of those? Well, that would also be compromised. Chronic diseases can also prevail due to lack of sleep. For instance insulin levels fluctuate, and blood pressure gets higher within 24 hours of sleeplessness, leading to diabetes and heart problems.

"But isn't this a book about our diet and nutrition?"

I am glad you asked, my friend. You see, your whole body is connected. The skeletal system is connected with the muscular system, the cardiovascular system is connected with the endocrine system, similarly the nervous system

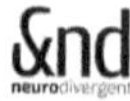

is also connected to the digestive system. I'm not going to bore you with a biology lecture on how these systems are connected, but I am going to talk about the link between sleep and diet, and how sleeplessness leads to obesity. It's quite simple actually – when you don't get enough sleep, your body increases the levels of cortisol and ghrelin. Meanwhile, leptin levels are decreased. Ghrelin is a hormone that is responsible for increased hunger, and leptin is the exact opposite of that. I am sure from here on, you can do the math as well. Increased hunger due to less sleep will eventually lead to weight gain and (if prolonged on a long-term basis) obesity.

The Quality Quotient

In 1964, a researcher named Hammond studied the importance of the quality of sleep where he explored insomnia in men. In his research, there wasn't a clear-cut definition for insomnia, but he did report that "not feeling refreshed after sleeping" can be considered as a symptom of insomnia. After this, many studies were conducted to determine more about insomnia and sleep patterns.

Sleep quality is different for different cultures all across the world. Other than that, the factors affecting the quality of sleep are delayed bedtime, varying family lifestyle, delayed waking up, and most important of all, screen time. Yes you heard that right. Even if you sleep for 8 hours a day, using too much screen in your day is going to give you a poor quality sleep.

At present there is no proper or official definition than can assess the quality of sleep, but there is a worldwide scale known as the Pittsburgh Sleep Quality Index (PSQI) which reveals the sleep quality on workdays only. However, one simple factor can assess sleep quality: the deviation from your optimal sleep. If you're waking up more frequently, or are getting disturbed easily during the night, this means that

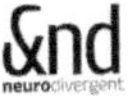

you're deviating from your optimal sleep pattern, and hence your sleep quality is reduced.

"But – "

Yes I am coming onto the dietary aspect of sleep duration. You need to learn to have some patience, my friend. Delayed mealtimes, and skipping breakfast have a direct effect on sleep quality. And the evidence for these is all there in the research articles. Poor sleep quality, such as experiencing frequent awakenings or disturbances during the night, can disrupt the body's natural circadian rhythm and affect various physiological processes, including appetite regulation. Sleep quality also change the levels of ghrelin and leptin, ghrelin is often referred to as the "hunger hormone," and increases appetite, while leptin is known as the "satiety hormone," and helps regulate feelings of fullness, causing changes in the appetite. And you know the drill – it leads to obesity.

The Consistency Quotient

Having a regular, consistent sleep will have so many positive influences on your body like weight maintenance, lower risks of chronic diseases, your mood improves, and so does your judgement. But does sleeping on a proper schedule really that important? Of course it is! Your body has its 'biological clock' which runs according to the pattern of daylight and helps regulate your sleep consistency naturally. This is why when it's the day, you need to remain active and work, and when it's nighttime, you need to have your sleep. That is also why it gets difficult for you to maintain your health when you're working the night shift, and / or changed a time zone (jet lag).

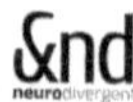

The Master Architect of Your Body's Repair and Renewal

You might often think that after a whole busy day, your brain needs some rest. And so, when you sleep, your brain gets its 'down time'. The concept is totally false. Our brain is working even during the night, while we're sleeping. Dr. Maiken Nedergaard, from the University of Rochester explained that sleep helps to prepare your brain for learning, remembering and creating. Moreover, while we're sleeping, the brain gets rid of some of the toxins using its drainage system. Her team had worked on mice and deduced that the drainage system removed a protein connected with Alzheimer's disease from the brain, and these toxins were removed faster while the mice were asleep.

You need to take care of your sleep patterns because there are some repairing functions that work best while you're asleep. It's when our muscles grow, our tissues repair, and our hormones regulate. So, when you're skipping out on sleep, don't be surprised when you find yourself feeling sluggish, weak, and prone to all sorts of health problems. Let's not forget about the incredible impact sleep has on our cognitive function. When you snooze, your brain is hard at work, consolidating memories, processing information, and sharpening your mental faculties. So, if you think you can pull an all-nighter and still function like a genius, think again. 'How' is the golden question here. Let me share some tips with you which can help you improve your sleep quantity, quality and consistency:

- Get some exercise everyday but not near to your bedtime.
- Create a sleep schedule: go to bed and wake up at the same time every day.
- Go outside and try to get some sunlight for half an hour.

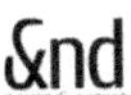

- Avoid nicotine and caffeine as they may keep you awake for a few hours.
- Avoid alcohol consumption as it prevents restorative sleep.
- Limit electronics before bedtime as the light from the screen keeps your brain active because it mistakes it for daylight. Try reading a book instead.
- Don't lie in bed awake. If you find it difficult to sleep after 20 minutes, try to do something that'll relax you.
- Keep a good and relaxing sleeping environment. Dim the lights, get rid of any annoying sounds, set the temperature of the room, keep your phone away.
- If nothing from the above mentioned tips helped you then you need to see a health care provider.
- If you have any kind of sleep disorder, like insomnia, then therapy and medication can really help you.

Sleep is not some optional extra in life, it is a non-negotiable, fundamental necessity for your overall health and well-being. It's time to wake up (pun intended) so quit fooling yourself and start giving sleep the respect it deserves. Establish a routine, create a cozy sleep haven, and for heaven's sake, put down those glowing screens before bed. Your body and mind will thank you.

"But Muneeba, my life is such a mess and it's stressing me out." Hey! Relax. I get how your life might be a mess right now, but there are ways to manage that too.

Cortisol and Calories

The connection between stress and diet is real. Stress is an unwelcome guest in your life, and it has a knack for wreaking havoc on your eating habits. When stress strikes, it's like a neon sign flashing *"emotional eating"* in bold, obnoxious letters. Suddenly, that perfectly planned balanced meal goes out the

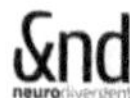

window, and you find solace in the comforting arms of greasy fast food, sugary treats, and all the oh-so-tempting junk. It has a way of convincing us, like a manipulative friend whispering, "Go ahead, indulge. You deserve it. It'll make you feel better." Yeah, right!

And let's not forget about those cravings. Stress has this uncanny ability to transform us into bottomless pits of hunger, yearning for all the wrong things. Suddenly, we're reaching for the nearest bag of chips, pint of ice cream, or that guilty pleasure chocolate bar that promises to make all our worries disappear. Spoiler alert: it won't.

The odyssey doesn't end here, stress doesn't just mess with your cravings; it messes with your bodies too. It's like a tornado tearing through your metabolism, leaving chaos and calorie retention in its wake. Stress hormones throw our bodies into survival mode, holding onto every ounce of fat like it's a precious life raft. It's like your body's saying, "Hey, let's add some extra padding to deal with all this stress, because that's exactly what we need, right?" And let's not overlook the emotional rollercoaster that stress takes us on. One minute we're drowning in deadlines and to-do lists, the next we're drowning our sorrows in a tub of ice cream. Emotional eating becomes the norm, as if food were the magic solution to all our problems. Spoiler alert number two: it's not.

And just like that you are caught in this frustrating cycle. Your mind, a mess. You're getting tricked by to sabotage all those efforts you made to maintain a healthy diet. But don't you worry, there's still hope for you.

Awareness is the first step. Next, find healthier outlets for your emotions, like exercise, meditation, or even a good old-fashioned venting session. Surround yourself with a support

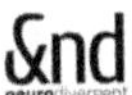

system that understands the struggles and can lend a listening ear or a helping hand.

Okay, let's do a calming exercise. Stand up, and follow the following steps:

- Find a quiet place, with minimum distractions. Dim the light and play some soothing music.
- Wear something comfortable that allows you to move freely.
- Start taking deep slow breaths. Inhale through your nose and exhale through your mouth.
- Gently stretch your body muscles by various yoga poses like the Child's pose, standing-forward-bent pose, legs-up-the-wall pose.
- Incorporate mindfulness by focusing on the sensations in your body, on the rhythm of your breathing. Feel the stretch and for a moment just think of the present, blocking out all worries from your mind.
- End with relaxation through the Corpse Pose. Lie down on your back, close your eyes, and allow your body to fully relax and soak in the benefits of your practice.

Do you feel lighter? I bet you do. Just remember, you are in control. Stress may try to pull the strings, but you have the power to resist its temptations. It may not be easy, and there may be slip-ups along the way, but don't let stress win this battle. Take charge of your diet, kick stress to the curb, and show that annoying little monster who's boss.

So, next time stress comes knocking, take a deep breath, find healthier alternatives, and give stress the sassy eyeroll it deserves. You've got this, and nothing, not even stress, can stand in your way.

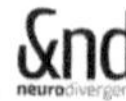

CHAPTER
8

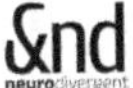

Mind Over Munch: Rewriting the Script

We've come a long way in our exploration of healthy living, tackling topics like myths, diet cultures, stress, sleep, and their impact on our bodies. But there's one critical aspect we haven't yet delved into: the role of beliefs and mindset. Yes, you heard it right—those sneaky little thoughts and attitudes that can either propel us towards success or drag us down into a pit of frustration. You need to get ready to challenge some of the most stubborn beliefs about food and exercise because that's exactly what we're going to do.

Beliefs and mindset not only act as a hinderance towards optimal heath care, but a particular set of beliefs can deceive you and keep you in denial. Let me elaborate using the simplest of examples; if you know someone who is a smoker, you'd realize that they most probably do not really believe in the harms of smoking. Even if they do believe that smoking causes problems in their body, they would always be in denial of the intensity or severity of the harmful effects that smoking has on them. The hindrance here is their perception. Similarly, if you are allergic to gluten, and you perceive it as a mild irritation, you might not avoid gluten that seriously and will most probably continue to suffer. Your culture, your traditions, your religion, your perceptions, all of these play the biggest role in your health.

From Heritage to Habits

A culture doesn't just consist of customs and traditions, it includes values, habits and attitudes as well. These are learned

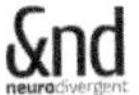

habits and values that have been adapted and acquired since childhood and most of these values are not deliberately taught, yet they run deep into our subconsciousness, affecting our life decisions.

Do you know that some cultures believe the 'R' rule for shellfish which is all about eating shellfish in the months that have an R in their names. Basically all the months of the year excluding May, June, July and August. This belief is justified by the red tide and spawning season. During breeding season certain toxins are produced in the bodies of these fish and shellfish poisoning can do terrible things to the human body. Whether this is a myth or not, it depends what culture you're asking. I don't want to go through the myth busting cycle again. Don't get me wrong, I love to debunk some myths and misconceptions. Something about telling the other person that they're wrong is just so satisfying (kidding, obviously). But what my rhetorical question actually meant was that I have explained and cleared up some of the most common misconceptions in the previous chapters. But the gravity of the situation is evident from the firm beliefs and blind following.

Talking about firm beliefs, I have to mention how much a culture has an impact on our eating habits. *"If it is on the table, do not ask for the salt and pepper,"* says the Portuguese. It probably means that the chef's pride is on the line. If a salt and pepper shaker is not provided to you, it means that you must like the exact amount of salt and pepper that the cook added. *"Never ask for cheese if it is not offered,"* says the Italians. Who knew Italians would be so defensive about cheese on their pizzas. *"Bread is not meant to be eaten as an appetizer,"* says the French. It's supposed to be eaten with the meal, not before it. The French also believe that there should be no money talk at mealtime, so if you're in a restaurant, do not talk about splitting the bills. Let one person bear the burden. *"Never stick your chopsticks upright in your rice,"* says the Japanese, because

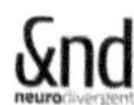

this practice is done at funerals. The Japanese also want you to *"slurp your food"* as they believe it enhances the flavors and also pays some sort of respect to the chef. Speaking of respect, some Inuit cultures of Canada believe that *"farting after a meal"* is a sign of respect too. It shows that you are thankful for your meal, but my advice here – do not mix these two: food and farts. South Koreans believe, *"no one should take a bite of the food until the oldest person there takes a bite,"* as a matter of fact, join your eating pace with them while you're at it and make sure you don't finish earlier or later than them. Throughout the Middle East, it is believed to *"eat with your right hand,"* and the logic behind this is that the right hand is for eating and left hand is for 'cleaning'. Whereas the Chinese believe that *"no hands are needed at all,"* and a knife and fork is expected to be used, no matter you're eating a pizza or fries. And on the contrary, the Mexicans say, *"do not eat tacos using a fork and knife,"* and this is understandable. It just seems silly to try to eat tacos with utensils. However, in Thailand, you're not allowed to *"put food in your mouth using a fork,"* it is only meant for helping the food into a spoon.

Almost all of these cultural norms are neither directly affecting your health, nor are they harmful for others around you (maybe except the one about the farts). Such kinds of beliefs that have a logic behind them generated by their heritage are personal, and I respect those, I really do. I mean, I also eat with my right hand, and never use utensils for tacos. Some of the cultural beliefs are actually beneficial, for instance elderly ladies would ask their daughters or daughters-in-law to drink sauerkraut juice just so they can detect whether they're pregnant or not. If the girls get sick after drinking it, they're pregnant, otherwise not. How is this beneficial? Well, sauerkraut juice is really good for pregnant women, so all those ladies who give out sauerkraut juice as a test, they're making their girls healthier.

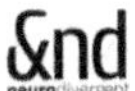

But there are some cultural norms that are just crazy. When I was a kid, I used to hang out at a friend's house a lot. Her grandmother had some crazy cultural beliefs which she used to inflict upon my friend's mother, for instance when we cut off the tips of the cucumbers and rub them , a white foamy stuff appears. It's the poison and that's how you get rid of it. Once told us that placing a hot potato on my head will cure my headache. Seeing the white foamy poison being washed away regularly made me think she is right, about both of these beliefs. Growing up, I realized that's not how it works but a part of me still feels relieved from a migraine after eating salty potato chips. I know, it's probably the salt that helps my nausea. But what can I say, cultural beliefs have the capability to dig its claws into your brain.

It's important to note that food myths can originate from various cultures or belief systems and may not be specific to a single one. The myths mentioned above are not necessarily tied to a particular culture or belief system. They are common misconceptions that can be found in different societies or propagated by individuals regardless of their cultural background. It's crucial to approach food myths with a critical mindset and rely on scientific evidence rather than attributing them solely to a specific culture or belief system.

The Healthy Lens: Shifting Perspectives on Wellness

Perception always plays a vital role when we want to categorize what's healthy and what isn't. For instance, it has been demonstrated quite often through surveys and research that people can live quite a healthy life despite their health and nutrition being inadequate according to Western standards. Which basically means that if you are considered as unhealthy in America, you are probably healthy in the Middle East.

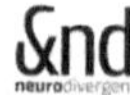

This varying perception might be either because it's possible that people may eat a nutrition-dense part of a plant or an animal that some communities discard as waste material, or because that particular community has adapted to thee food they eat, mainly prevailing due to their socioeconomic statuses. This remind us that it is not okay to use the same set of standards for industrialized societies and underdeveloped societies. In short, we need to change our perceptions about food items, and health standards when it comes to different regions of the world. You might wonder why there is such a difference in awareness regarding diet and nutrition among different areas of the world. Let me share a research conducted for this particular question. Spoiler alert: Health care professionals is the answer. Have a look:

The GP's Prescription for Wellness – Health Starts Here

Did you know that the practice done by the general practitioners in various countries has a huge impact on our belief systems? There are research articles and surveys conducted about this and let me tell you, it is a lot serious than it sounds.

An article provided evidence that the knowledge and training of the general practitioners needs to be upgraded to evidence-based programs, interventions and easy-to-use tools in order to make their patient believe how important diet and physical activity are for weight management.

That particular study was conducted in European countries and the question that the researchers asked was about the discussion regarding lifestyle changes between them and their GP. Some patients stated that they really needed to change their eating habits and the amount of physical activity in a day. While others explained how they will keep this lifestyle modification need in mind. However, the researchers had an idea that their responses might not be a hundred percent

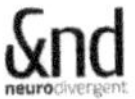

true since it seemed like they may have provided them with "socially desirable" answers.

The interesting factor in this research was the times when the GP initiated this particular discussion themselves. Only half of the patients reported that the general practitioners talked about lifestyle modification. It's quite alarming. You see, when you visit a general practitioners, he or she needs to know about your habits and must recommend modifications in your routine that will definitely be for the sake of your health, which is exactly the reason why you went to the GP in the first place. If this practice is not being done, then the patients might not receive the proper medical care and attention that they require.

The study did not discover the reason for why GPs do not emphasize on such therapies and treatments, but it can only be speculated that the advice for nutrition and physical activity is not provided for the sole purpose of being too time consuming. It is often difficult to evaluate the effectiveness of these said lifestyle changes as well. Moreover, it is also quite possible that these GPs and healthcare providers might not be reimbursed. On top of that, the general practitioners believed that they should definitely advice the patient regarding prevention and health promotion activities, but it wasn't clear whether the GPs did that in regard to the eating habits and the physical activities (or lack thereof).

Holy Health

Religious beliefs are concrete. Such beliefs are based on your consciousness and that's why these are the strongest. Take the example of Muslim people and how they practice fasting in their Holy month of Ramadan. My high school best friend was a Muslim and trust me when I say this, it is not possible for a Muslim of strong faith to break his or her fast before

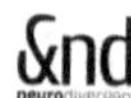

the allotted time, no matter how thirsty and hungry they are. There were so many ways that all of us friends tried to tempt Omar, but he was one spiritually strong 16 year old. Of course I do realize that we might not have been as respectful as needed. But the point is that he never gave in. Muslims have a fixed time for starting their fast, and a fixed time of breaking it – from dawn till dusk – and they don't consume neither food nor water.

Not only mealtimes, but also the type of food to be consumed is also determined by religion. For example Jews and Muslims do not eat pork but they can eat other kinds of meat only if it has been properly sacrificed according to their religious laws, Hindus are against killing or eating cattle. Mexican Indians will prefer a bad crop of corn over a good crop of any other plant because their attitude towards corn is quite religious.

Some people may also become vegetarians due to religious beliefs. Others might turn towards the vegetarian life just because of the thought that plant foods have a superior virtue. While others prefer vegetables only because they dislike other food options – and that's their perception and attitude towards that food product. Some communities believe in eating only seasonal fruits and vegetables which is why they don't believe in storing or preserving them. I have no such comment on whether these religious beliefs make sense or not, but the truth is that the people following the religion believe in these food limitations with all their hearts.

Attitude Reset

It's not just the religion, customs, preferences and perceptions, but also the attitude that decides for us what to eat, what's healthy, when to eat and how to eat. It's all about the mind and let's just face it: your mind can be your greatest ally or your fiercest foe. The only belief system or school of thought

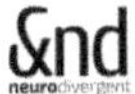

I am against is the belief that you'll never be able to stick to a healthy diet, or that you're inherently lazy. Such deeply ingrained negative beliefs can sabotage your progress. Don't worry, we've all been there at a point in our lives, battling with negative self-talk, doubting our abilities, and succumbing to self-sabotage.

This book had always been about challenging those self-limiting thoughts head-on by realizing the importance of cultivating a positive mindset and banishing those limiting beliefs that hold you back from achieving your health goals.

Let's face it: it's time to break free from this self-imposed mental prison.

Hey, You! Be Kind to Yourself and Take Care

Sarah's journey never quite ends. She goes through a constant struggle. Sometimes she gives up, and after a while she dusts herself off and picks herself up. In the quest for a healthier lifestyle, she forget one crucial ingredient: self-compassion. Until she was told that the path to lasting change isn't paved with punishment and self-criticism but with kindness and understanding. Self-compassion was a game-changer when it came to how Sarah handle food and exercise. It was all about treating herself with love and acceptance, embracing her strengths and imperfections.

When it comes to food, self-compassion means saying farewell to guilt and shame. No more beating yourself up for enjoying a treat or going off your usual eating plan. You should always give yourself some room for mistakes and learn to find balance and moderation. Nourishing your body isn't just about the nutrients, it's about feeding your souls with joy and pleasure. It's a complete process: you savor your meals, listen to your

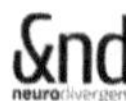

body, and make choices that make you feel good inside and out.

And exercise? Well, it's never about fixing your body. It's more like an act of self-care and self-love. No more forcing yourself into strict workout routines that feel like a chore. Instead, focus on activities that light you up, make you feel alive, and energized. Self-compassion should remind you that rest and recovery are just as important as getting our sweat on. You listen to your body and find the balance that suits you. To find that balance, you have got to be honest with yourself. Honor your needs, whether it's about eliminating a food group that is not good for you, or simply taking a break. Ditch the idea of perfection and focus on progress and growth.

It's like saying, "Hey, I deserve love and care just as I am!"

Embrace the power of your mind and embark on a journey of self-discovery and empowerment. Just remember, you have the ability to reshape your beliefs, transform your mindset, and create a thriving, joyful, and sustainable approach to food and exercise. The choice is yours, so let's break free and live our healthiest lives yet.

I feel like singing a song.

> "Say what you wanna say
> And let the words fall out
> Honestly, I wanna see you be brave"
> *–"Brave" by Sara Bareilles*

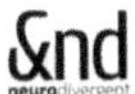

As we wrap up this journey, let's not forget the power of simplicity. Often, the most obvious things are the easiest to overlook. So here's a cheeky twist, a delicious surprise at the end of our feast. Don't be mad at me when I say, this entire book could be boiled down to a catchy, four-word jingle:

Calories in, Calories out.

Yes, you heard it right! This simple, yet profound mantra holds the essence of our voyage into the world of nutrition. As you chart your own course to wellbeing, let these four words be your compass, guiding you through the maze of food choices and diet decisions. Remember, it's all about balance. Here's to you, bravely setting sail on your nutrition journey!

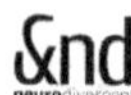